The Baby Voyage

An Adventure in

Maternity Leave Abroad

Erick and Kasey Prato

Contents

Reference Maps

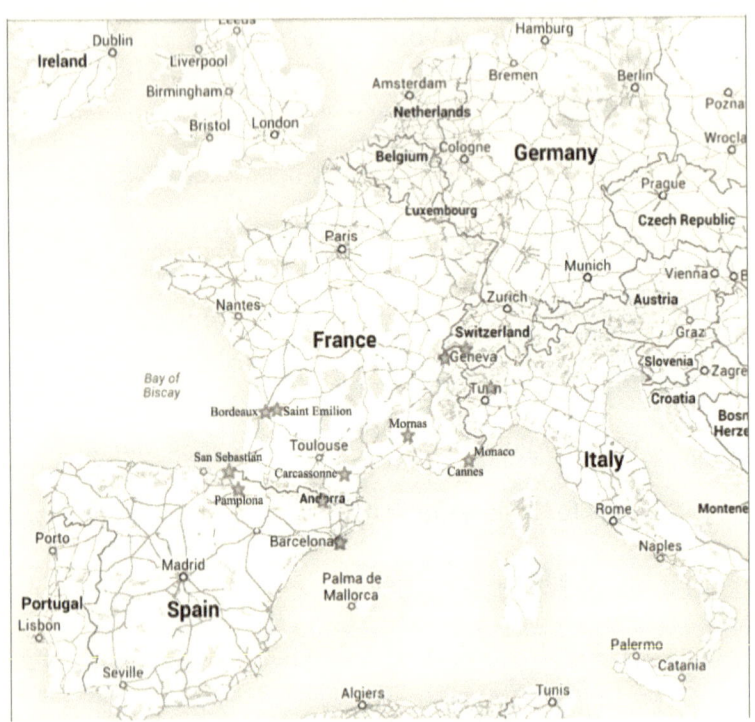

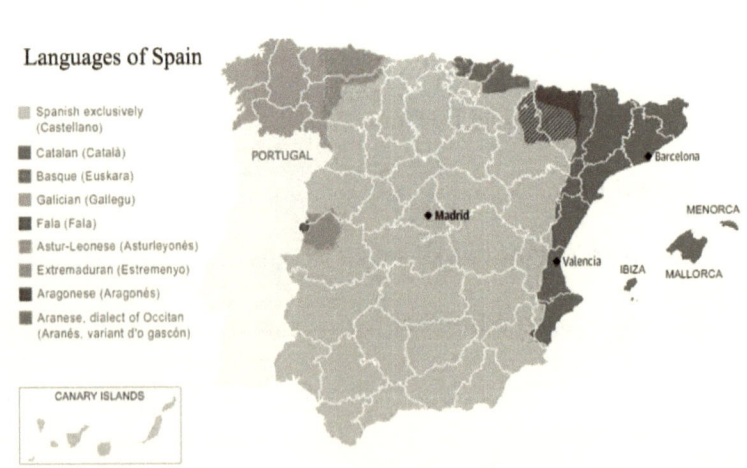

Languages of Spain

- Spanish exclusively (Castellano)
- Catalan (Català)
- Basque (Euskara)
- Galician (Gallegu)
- Fala (Fala)
- Astur-Leonese (Asturleyonés)
- Extremaduran (Estremenyo)
- Aragonese (Aragonés)
- Aranese, dialect of Occitan (Aranés, variant d'o gascón)

Introduction

When we were expecting our first child in 2010, we made the unconventional decision to leave our home in Florida and travel to Barcelona, Spain, a city we had previously visited for only a few days on our honeymoon, for the birth of our daughter and to spend the duration of a three month maternity leave. We made this decision for a myriad of reasons which are detailed in the following pages, but from the planning stages to our homecoming, the experience turned out to be an even bigger adventure than we had bargained for filled with plenty of surprises and all the thrills and perils of international travel, immersion in a new culture and language and, of course, being first time parents!

As this was a truly transformative time in the life of our family, we hoped to put into writing for our children the values and dreams which led us to go on *The Baby Voyage* and to where we are in our lives today as we seek to continue living a more deliberate life and to dare to question and challenge the assumptions we all make about what is possible by always asking, "What would it take?" That is, what would it take to turn our dreams into goals so that we might then dedicate our time and effort to making those dreams our reality.

The Baby Voyage is written in both of our voices and each chapter is preceded by a small male or female figure to let you know who is talking. We hope you enjoy our story.

Here We Go

"No, no! The adventures first, explanations take such a dreadful time." — Lewis Carroll, Alice's Adventures in Wonderland & Through the Looking-Glass

That night, the airplane bathroom seemed even smaller than usual. But then again, at thirty-five weeks pregnant, everything had gotten to be a tight fit. Thankfully, I had become proficient at the quick run to the ladies' room. But just as I was beginning to struggle with my flight-recommended, ultra-super-support, pregnant-lady pantyhose, the pilot came over the intercom:

> Good evening Ladies and Gentleman. This is your Captain speaking. Sorry for the interruption, but it looks like we might have an—ummm—maintenance problem. We are going to need to turn around and head back to Atlanta. Sorry for the inconvenience, but it is just not the kind of thing—you know—that you really want while you're flying over the North Atlantic at night.

These were not exactly the reassuring words we had wanted to hear from our pilot after almost two hours in the air on our flight to Europe. I thought to myself, he is kidding, right? I worked my way out of the bathroom and back to my seat. No punchline yet from the cockpit and absolutely no attempt to assuage the growing concerns of the passengers. According to my husband, Erick, who is fluent in Spanish, the Spanish speaking flight attendant was, however, doing a markedly better public relations job. Without any further explanation on the nature of the "problem," after few minutes, the pilot again:

> Sorry for another interruption, but if you look out the windows you may see a stream coming off the wings. It is nothing to worry about, folks; it is just jet fuel. It is going to be pretty *spectacular* though.

Once, when Erick and I were boarding a flight to South Carolina (my home state), he started discussing with me how "primitive" airplanes really are. I advised him that as far as I was concerned, at that moment, the airplane I was on was the most technologically advanced machine in human history. Not that I am a particularly nervous flyer, but much like the term "primitive," "spectacular" is not a word I want used to describe any in-flight event.

Back on our red-eye flight to Spain, due to the increasing discrepancy between the English and Spanish accounts coming from the cockpit, while half of the plane's passengers looked reasonably calm and reassured, the non-Spanish speaking passengers were on the verge of panic. Without providing further specifics, the pilot turned the plane away from our long-awaited destination, and back toward Hartsfield-Jackson Atlanta International. Over three hours into the flight and with us now making backward progress, the pilot:

> Hello again, folks. We need to talk about this landing. (I was hopeful for a moment that the Spanish translator might give this pep talk—but no.) It looks like we are going to need the *whole* runway. Please be sure your seatbelts are fastened.

And with that admonition, down we went; indeed coming to a halt just at the tip of the airport runway. We all deplaned, without ever knowing the true nature and extent of our peril, but safe and relieved to be free from the potentially spectacular.

Having been set back several hours, I was as anxious as ever to get going. After all, this trip had been a long time in the making. Blissfully, just before 11:00 p.m., we were onboard a new plane (unfortunately with the same pilot) and back in the air. Having begun our journey more than 12 hours before in Florida, I was exhausted, in need of yet another bathroom break and full of excitement and anticipation.

First Things First

The Beginning of a Dream

"The future is something which everyone reaches at the rate of sixty minutes an hour, whatever he does, whoever he is."
— C.S. Lewis

When I was five years old, my parents took my older brother and me to Walt Disney World. I was instantly drawn to the popular "Small World" ride. So much so, that after several trips around the Small World river, which takes visitors on a boat ride through hundreds of dancing dolls dressed in traditional clothing from all over the world, when my parents let me throw a penny into the water to make a wish, I wished to ride just one more time! To my ten-year-old brother's extreme annoyance, off we went again. I am fairly sure that my parents assumed that as a little girl, I was interested in the dolls, the dancing and the music. I have always loved to dance, but I think the real attraction for me was the journey. We got to go around the entire world on that little boat and I loved it! To me it seemed magical. Not to worry, my brother did eventually make it to Space Mountain and my parents (I hope) were able to get that song out of their heads (thank you both), but I had already caught the travel bug and it has never gone away.

Today, I love to travel, to try new things and meet new and interesting people. I can also be restless and enjoy just "being on the go." For many years, I wished that I had studied or lived abroad and that I had committed myself to learning a new language. I regretted not having done so in college when time was easy and my commitments few, but as a 30-year-old, married, practicing attorney who wanted a family, time seemed much more scarce. But still, I longed for the chance and daydreamed about ways to do it. I met Erick in Fort Lauderdale in the fall of 2005, and we were married in April 2008. We knew that we wanted children within a few years and Erick shared my passion for learning and exploring. And, as luck would have it, Erick had a very compatible dream.

As I mentioned, I had always wanted to master a second language. Unfortunately, my high school and college Spanish left me without the fluency I dreamed of, and regrettably, although I had traveled internationally, I did not study abroad, nor did I spend the time necessary for real immersion. The benefits of learning a new language are innumerable and I had always had the desire, but now I had additional leverage. My firstborn child was on the way and I wanted to help her be bilingual from day one. Since Erick already spoke Spanish, many said that he could just teach our children, but from the experiences of countless friends and acquaintances, it is much easier if both parents are onboard and involved. But language goals aside, I longed to experience life in another culture, to break out of our day-to-day and maybe even return to see our own lives in a new light.

When I was in the second grade, my family moved in the middle of the school year. I particularly remember one of my first classes when the teacher asked the class to draw our flag. I thought it was an easy assignment until I began to struggle drawing the stars in the middle of the flag. I looked around to see how my classmates were doing it. To my surprise, the kids next to me did not have the yellow, blue and red stripes that I expected. I got nervous thinking that I had misunderstood the teacher. Since I was new, maybe the other kids knew something I did not. As I was wondering about this, I finally decided to stand up and look at what the kids sitting in front and behind me were doing. The teacher did not like this and had me back in my seat before I could get a good peek. The time ran out and I still had not finished my stars. As she started collecting the drawings, I noticed that less than half of the class had drawn the same flag. There were all kinds. I did not understand how so many kids could have such different drawings for the same assignment, and thought maybe only some of us got it right. Only much later did I realize what happened that day. Many of these kids' parents were foreign.

Having been born in Venezuela, a leading oil producing nation, at a time when the country's economy was booming (peaking in the 1970s) and attracting immigrants from all over the world, I became accustomed to having friends that spoke other languages at home. I moved to the United States myself when I was 20 years old and had to face all of the challenges associated with learning a new language and adapting to a new culture. Like most people, as I matured and started planning to have a family, I wanted to give my children the things and opportunities I did not have as a child. I wanted them to grow up speaking several languages and being comfortable in different cultures. Growing up in the United States, my children would be native English speakers and I could teach them Spanish at home. They would not have a foreign accent in either language. Friends would tell me that I could teach my children the "best of both worlds" and that way they would "have it all" like I wanted. However, I knew that there was much more than two languages and two countries, so why not give them access to at least another culture and another language? Since English and Spanish were covered, and although I love Italian, French seemed to me like the next most practical international language. Now, I just needed to move to France and live there long enough with them to learn the language and assimilate the culture before coming back to the U.S.

Moving to another country has many challenges even in the best of circumstances and the idea of going through it again in my late twenties was just daunting. I kept thinking there had to be a better way. I would joke that all I needed to do was to find a wonderful French woman already living in the U.S., hope that she would find me irresistible, fall in love, get married, have children and live happily ever after. We could teach our children Spanish and French at home in addition to English. A great start in an increasingly flatter, and more multicultural and globalized world, I thought. My dream for my children did not seem any more attainable, though, since I wasn't actually looking for such a woman, but I kept dreaming.

Finding the woman I wanted to marry and have children with turned out to be more difficult than I expected (French speaking or not). I feared that it would also be hard to find someone likeminded who would share my dreams. As I turned 30, while going to church in Fort Lauderdale, I met Kasey. She was very intelligent, curious, kind, patient and attractive. She was open-minded, a great dancer, liked to travel and for some inexplicable reason, was attracted to me. She turned out to be everything I could hope for in a woman and more (even though she didn't speak French). Kasey actually had to convince me that she really liked me, including my "crazy" dreams (I would later joke with her that maybe she wasn't so smart after all). After we got married, when friends started asking about our family plans, I would smile and say that I wanted to have eight children and for each of them to be born in a different country (you can see how over time my dream had continued to evolve). In response to their inquisitive looks, Kasey would laugh. I don't think that even Kasey realized I wasn't completely joking.

The Big Idea

*"All the forces in the world are not so powerful
as an idea whose time has come." — Victor Hugo*

When Erick and I started planning a family and he told me about his dreams for our children, which were in tune with my own, we began to discuss our options for reaching our goals. We were both eager to begin the process of immersing ourselves and our children in another language and culture and often dreamed together about how and when we might get started. Eventually, after much consideration, and afraid to put off our dreams any longer, we established the Big Idea—the long and short of which was that we would start this process for our children at the very beginning. That is, when I got pregnant, I would give birth and we would spend my maternity leave *abroad*! But before we could board the plane and *The Baby Voyage* could really begin, there were obviously some details to work out. Let's answer the most burning question first: Why during maternity leave?

With both Erick and I working full-time and intending to continue doing so for the foreseeable future, maternity leave was essentially the only time I could take several months off from work and keep my job. To be clear, we are not exactly hippies (or independently wealthy) and both felt we were a little past the time for backpacking through Europe, even if we had ever been so inclined. We wanted and intended to return to our lives and jobs in the U.S. after our trip. As for Erick, he was also eligible for three months unpaid leave as a new father under the Family Medical Leave Act. He will fill in the details about his challenges, but as two busy working professionals, maternity leave, although counterintuitive for some, seemed just the right time for us to strike out and begin this adventure.

Since this trip would involve my pregnancy and our first child, it would not be the kind of travel where we could just improvise as we had done many times in the past. As the time neared when we hoped to get pregnant, we needed to ensure that we had a sound plan to execute what was no longer just our *dream* but our *goal*.

International travel is one of my passions. Instead of resting from a busy life, I seek adventure away from the routine. I much prefer to travel without tour guides or package arrangements, and love to get around on my own trying different methods of transportation whenever possible. This allows me to really get away from everything that is familiar to me and have the experience of adventure and discovery that I seek in a trip. There is nothing like exploring on my own, without feeling limited to do what some travel agency decided was relevant. Being flexible, one can also save a lot of money. I love talking with the locals anywhere I go and one can always find people eager to tell you about themselves, their hometowns, favorite foods, traditions, and so on and they let you know about the surprising places that most tourists don't ever hear about. Locals also share a wealth of information on what it is like to actually live in their town, what they love and what they don't, and with everything from education, to the cost of living and local politics, I find it all fascinating.

By the time Kasey and I were married and ready to start our family, we had already taken several international trips together. I planned each trip myself and was able to make all the arrangements online, from the transportation to booking the hotels. I would put all the details in a spreadsheet and show them to Kasey before committing any money. Kasey was always excited to go anywhere and enjoyed every trip—even when I got us lost misreading a map, booked a bad hotel or looked stupid asking people all kinds of disparate questions about anything I considered unusual.

For our honeymoon, we went to Europe. We visited a high school friend of mine that was now living in Madrid, Spain (where his parents had been born). From there, we went to Barcelona for three days and then on to Italy and Greece, where my brother lived at the time (having married a Greek-Venezuelan). Since I planned this trip on my own, I indulged my fascination for different modes of transportation and we took everything from planes, to trains, boats, taxis, subways—you name it. Kasey said that it was a bit like being on the Amazing Race and I admit that I may have tried to do a little too much. However, we still enjoyed ourselves very much and we learned what our ideal speed was. The more we traveled, the more comfortable we felt in foreign places and the more we talked about life overseas and how we wished we spoke other languages. These trips also really prepared us for our maternity leave adventure since we had already gotten to know each other, not only as husband and wife, but also as travel partners, which can sometimes be a whole different story.

What Would it Take?

"If one advances confidently in the direction of his dreams, and endeavors to live the life which he has imagined, he will meet with a success unexpected in common hours. He will put some things behind, will pass an invisible boundary; new, universal, and more liberal laws will begin to establish themselves around and within him." — Henry David Thoreau, Walden

I like to think of myself as a realist and a rational person and I think that unfortunately, most dreams are just that—dreams. However, as we go through life and meet and read about remarkable people, it becomes evident that some dreams do become reality. I am of the opinion that we should invest a good amount of our mental energy challenging our preconceptions and realistically figuring out which of our dreams are attainable and which are simply too improbable.

For every dream I like to ask: "What would it take?" Rigorously and honestly answering this question can be a liberating and quite entertaining mental exercise. Either we will feel empowered to pursue our aspiration or we will at least stop lamenting not having fulfilled an impossible fantasy (such as in my case, traveling back in time to grow up speaking many languages or, for Kasey, becoming a Rockette).

The biggest obstacle to my dream of living in Europe long enough for me and my children to learn French had always been finding the woman willing to do it with me. Now that I had found in Kasey a willing and eager adventure partner with a similar but different dream, we just needed to work out a compromise.

Kasey wanted to live abroad, learn Spanish and raise bilingual children. I wanted to live in France and learn French along with my children. Kasey was open to the idea of going to any Spanish speaking country so, although we considered several different cities in Latin America, Spain was the obvious best compromise. It was in Europe, Kasey could learn Spanish there and I hoped that if we picked a city close enough to the French border, maybe I could study and practice French as well.

Once we answered the question, "What would it take?" and reached the conclusion that it was not impossible, we just needed to come up with ways to pursue it. The dream had been moved to the category of a goal. Once it became a goal, we tried to anticipate as many scenarios as possible, fully expecting surprises along the way. We remained flexible knowing that Kasey may not get pregnant when we hoped, once pregnant she may not be healthy enough to travel or that our job situations might change. Only God knew how things would actually happen for us. But barring any unforeseen circumstances, and with all the big questions answered, everything else was just logistics that we would eventually need to work out. As new parents-to-be we also, of course, had lots of questions anyway. For example, we even wondered if we could influence the gender of the baby before getting pregnant. Everything we read about that topic looked like voodoo to us, though, and we didn't care anyway (but it was fun to wonder).

When choosing the actual city, Barcelona was always our top contender. It is, in Kasey's words, a "real city" without being overwhelming. It has extraordinary architecture and history, it is vibrant and cosmopolitan, it has a great public transportation system and it is an international hub full of interesting activities in and around the city. It has beaches and pleasant weather year-round and is ideally located for travel enthusiasts like us with lots of other intriguing destinations within driving distance.

There were some issues though. While Spanish is widely spoken in Barcelona, the native language is actually Catalan. There are four official languages spoken in Spain, as well as several others. Catalan is a completely different language altogether, like French or Italian. Not even I as a native Spanish speaker can understand it. We were not sure if this fact would be an impediment to Kasey's learning Spanish.

Since Spanish acquisition was one of Kasey's main goals, we looked for alternatives and researched several other cities in Spain and Latin America, but it seemed that no place was just right. According to our research online, every other city we looked up seemed to have the "wrong" accent or had another native language that would impede one's learning. Language aside, we identified some other very important issues with other top contenders, such as: they were not by the beach (Kasey's problem), were too hot in the summer (a problem for me) or simply too far from France (also me). After much research, Barcelona remained our best choice. The more Kasey read about it, the more she liked it. It is less than two hours from France and I joked with Kasey that I would be crossing the border every weekend just to practice the French I would be learning while there. Having become an avid snowboarder while living in Denver, I also imagined myself hitting the slopes in the Pyrenees (also only a couple of hours away from Barcelona) at least once or twice. But given that our trip would be during the summer and that we would have a newborn baby, it was unlikely that I would be doing much snowboarding.

Family Matters

"Time will explain." — Jane Austen, Persuasion

Chief among my concerns for the trip was how my family would react to the news. I decided not to tell them until a few months prior to the planned departure date in June. I waited as long as I could to make sure the pregnancy was going well and that there would be no health concerns. I also wanted to have as many answers as possible for the questions I knew would come. Mom was first. I should say here that my entire family lives in South Carolina, a 12 hour drive from our home in Florida, so they were unlikely to have been present for the actual delivery even had we stayed in the U.S. Both of my parents were working and would probably only have been able to visit for a few days after our baby was born.

I gave Mom a call in the early spring to share the Big Idea. Mom, whose self-proclaimed goal is to find and reside in Mayberry from *The Andy Griffith Show*, is not really much of a traveler herself. She avoids flying whenever possible, preferring instead to load up the car with enough supplies for every conceivable contingency (full rack of clothes suitable for any occasion or weather emergency, coolers of food in case of famine in Florida, etc.).

Mom is also famous among my friends for her zealous and oft-repeated warnings: "Watch out for deer (we lived in rural S.C.), pickpockets on shore (in port cities anywhere other than The South), black ice on the road (you know you can never see it)," and so on. Suffice it to say, there would be concerns. Mom was driving when I called that evening and, in hindsight, I should have waited until she was home. I started out, "Mom, I have some news to share." Without missing a beat, Mom replied,

"Oh no, don't tell me you are planning to go to Egypt or something with the baby!" I guess we are not so unpredictable.

There are five stages of grief: (1) denial/isolation; (2) anger; (3) bargaining; (4) depression; and (5) acceptance. Mom flew right through the first two, briefly touching on denial, and made her way to stage three in record time. Within an hour, she was offering us cash not to do this. She even called back with a detailed payment plan. Acceptance was a *much* longer time coming. Sometime in August, after our daughter was born, Mom (sort of) began to appreciate our decision and I am pleased to note that she has since commented on many of the obvious benefits for our family. But that was not the case in the beginning.

I knew that Mom was not going to be wild about this idea, but I was not quite prepared for her reaction. According to the only eyewitness to the scene (my Mom) when she got home that night, she threw herself on the floor and *sobbed* at the thought that we would be out of the country for the birth of our first child. I think she cried partly because this would keep her from immediately seeing the baby and according to Mom, she needed to "imprint" herself on the baby right away. But I suspect the much stronger fear was that some unimaginably horrible thing would befall us in Spain and that we would surely regret this whole crazy business. For a few weeks following that conversation, Mom couldn't even talk to me about our plans. I think she did not want to condone our behavior. But eventually, as she realized we were serious and that we were really doing our homework in order to go, she became slightly more at peace (at least she started to pretend).

As I was traveling to South Carolina around Easter to visit my family, I waited to tell Dad in person (my parents are divorced). Going into this a little traumatized by Mom's reaction, I was not exactly sure what Dad would have to say, but I was more or less certain he would also be fairly lackluster in his support for this plan. Dad is certainly more inclined to travel and he knew that Erick and I "did things differently" but he was not expecting this. Erick and I were sitting with Dad on his screened-in porch overlooking the Tiger River at his house when we broke the news. Although what I said was that we were planning to have the baby in Spain and that we would return to the U.S. just two months later, his immediate reaction was to ask my stepmother, who had been out of the room, "Did you hear that? They are not going to let us see the baby." I did my best to calm that concern and explained that we intended to come for a visit in South Carolina within weeks of our return (which we did in October when our daughter was just two months old). Dad then asked us many of the same questions that we would hear often.

Dad may not have been the first person to mention *Them*, but he certainly gave the most curious response to our standard question, "Who?" For the uninitiated, *They* are the unknowable, omnipresent and all-mighty legion of gatekeepers dedicated to standing in your way and keeping you from realizing your dreams. Dad was but one of many who suggested that They were not going to let us do this. We posed the question, "Who are They?" to my father. Perhaps a little caught off-guard, but not one to be without an answer, he replied with certainty, "Obama." For the record, President Obama in no way interceded during this process either to hinder or facilitate our plans—presumably because he was busy with more pressing matters.

Mom, on the other hand, was really counting on Them to stop us. Surely some gatekeeper somewhere (a doctor, my employer, the insurance company, Erick's boss, the airline TSA agent, a Spanish immigration official, the clerk at Buy Buy Baby—*somebody*) would have the authority to end this madness. When Mom first heard the news, she also tried to enlist my big brother to help talk some sense into us. Surely he would have something to say. We shared the news with my brother over lunch that Easter weekend just after we arrived in South Carolina. Aside from a raised eyebrow of curiosity, and a laugh, he did not give Mom the reaction she was hoping for. My brother and his wife were also expecting their second child just five weeks after our daughter was due. A few months later, in an attempt to playfully antagonize Mom (and no doubt to one-up me), my brother announced that they would be having their baby girl in Rome! He was clearly not going to be of much help. In the end, they stuck with their plans to deliver in South Carolina and Mom was ultimately disappointed as we made it to Spain without my brother or any of Them standing in the way. Upon reading a draft of this book, however, Mom remarked that she would still like to hold Them accountable.

My family knew about my dream of living in Europe with my kids and learning other languages, however, they were surprised that I was really going to do it, that Spain would be the destination and mostly, that Kasey was onboard. My sister also lives in the U.S. and my younger brother has lived in the U.S., Greece and had recently moved to Australia. My parents still live in Venezuela and, from their point of view, they already expected their grandchildren to be born "abroad."

This does not mean that they were always onboard with the idea of international living though. When I was 19 years old, and told them about my plans to move to the U.S. within a year, they were adamantly against it. They did everything within their power to dissuade me and we had many fights about it for months. Apart from the one time when we had gone to Disney World when I was five years old, all they knew about the U.S. concerned the worst and most sensationalistic events they had seen on their local TV news along with the violence they had seen in American action movies. Much like all we had heard in the local U.S. news in the past few years about Spain had concerned the European debt crisis or the occasional reference to the bull fighting debate, with regard to their kids moving to the U.S., all my parents could think of was American involvement in wars, drug use, street gangs, AIDS, mass shootings and natural disasters.

As far as they knew, back in the early 90s (way before Chavez was elected) when I wanted to move to the U.S., Venezuela was still the richest, best country in the world as was evident from its large oil reserves, year-round spring weather and the foreigners from everywhere that had chosen it for a home. Just in the eight story building where they still live, we had neighbors from Holland, Spain, Portugal and Italy, among other nationalities. The national narrative was that the country was just going through a rough patch due to bad politicians. Venezuelans had never been immigrants and the idea of their children being the foreigners in the U.S. gave them chills, but nothing they did or said could dissuade me.

After I moved to the U.S. and my parents started coming to visit, they learned that there were many more positive things about the U.S. than what they had seen on TV. Now they think that it was a good thing that their children moved abroad and they knew that their grandkids would be born abroad too. As Kasey's Mom so eloquently described it when she was disappointed (yet again) to hear that my parents did not try to talk me out of having our daughter born in Spain: "They were already resigned to their fate."

They, Them and Others

"Don't waste your time with explanations; people only hear what they want to hear." — *Paulo Coelho*

As Kasey's pregnancy moved along, friends, coworkers, acquaintances and even passing strangers would congratulate us, show their excitement for us and then ask the usual questions: "How far along are you? Are you planning to find out the sex of the baby? Do you have a name? Is the nursery ready? When are you having the baby shower? In which hospital are you planning to give birth? Is your Mom coming to help?" We could not answer many of these casual questions without talking about our plans to go abroad.

Kasey is a more private person than I am, and since she expected many of these questions and anticipated that some people might react with surprise and doubt, she wanted to make sure she had good answers before she started sharing our plans. I, on the other hand, did not like the idea of not telling people until the last minute because keeping secrets makes me feel like I am doing something wrong. I was also so excited that I was eager to share our plans with everybody. Therefore, we agreed that I would tell my family, personal friends and coworkers and Kasey would tell her friends and family when she was ready. Since I started telling my friends and coworkers months before Kasey, I got to "discuss" the whole matter much longer than I was ready for and, as it turns out, I was not really prepared for what happened next.

At first, most people simply did not believe me, but after realizing that I was serious, close friends acted thoroughly disappointed and some were visibly upset at the idea that we would be having our first child overseas. Even coworkers and acquaintances that had no stake whatsoever in our lives reacted like we were about to commit a cardinal sin. The truth is it was comical to see completely random people react with such intensity to a personal decision that was completely inconsequential to them. I was expecting some of the usual skepticism when one makes an unconventional decision, and that close friends and, of course, Kasey's family in particular, would express concern. However, I was flabbergasted by the intensity of most people's reactions and that some seemed actually offended by our plans. Pretty soon, I found myself justifying our plans and discussing every conceivable scenario in excruciating detail. In retrospect, it is clear to me that Kasey's approach to wait as long as possible before telling anyone was much wiser.

Although I am focusing on the more distressed reactions here, to be clear, not everybody's reaction was negative. We did have a few friends that thought the idea of spending maternity leave abroad was just great. They congratulated us, got excited with us, asked many of the same questions (with curiosity instead of alarm) and joked about how envious they were and how they wished they had thought of it when they had their children, or wished that they had the courage to do it themselves. But as for the majority, after they realized that we were not joking about our plans, almost invariably the first question was: "Will They let you do that?" I found this question both amusing and perplexing and would usually reply with: "Who?" After a confused pause, I would get a response that started something like, "I don't know—you know—They," followed by at least one of the following answers (more often than not with frustration as though the answer was obvious and I was just being difficult): "the doctor, the hospital, the airline, the insurance company, Kasey's boss, my company, my boss, Kasey's Mom, Kasey's family, my Mom, Spain, the U.S. government!"

It seemed that whoever it was, from the doctor to the government, somebody must be able to stop two mature, financially independent, responsible, married adults from having their first baby in another country. This seemingly universal reaction made me wonder about how un-free some people must feel to make an unconventional or unusual decision, no matter how personal. I was utterly astonished by how many people were willing to relinquish personal freedom out of fear to the undefined, but all-powerful *They*.

After much speculation on my part and some less than pleasant discussions with a couple of my friends that had the strongest reactions, my conclusion was that after the initial surprise, they felt mostly annoyed and upset at my seemingly utter disregard for what They (aka: other people) would think or say. Once my question about the identity of the mysterious They was covered (or uncovered), some people would stop asking questions altogether. A few would not even dare to speak about the fearsome They openly. Others would alarmingly follow up with even more questions: "Will They let you bring the baby back? Will the baby be American? What about your home? Do they have a Babies "R" Us over there?"

There were a couple of instances in which people acted very nonchalantly, assuming that I was from Spain and that my family lived there or, interestingly enough, that I knew people who had done the same thing (therefore making it okay, I guess). When I clarified that neither was the case, they seemed equally shocked. But of all the questions we were asked, by far the most common was: "What about the *stuff*?" How were we going to take *everything* with us? I also found this question puzzling and would reply: "What stuff?" In response, I heard, "You know—all the things that the baby will *need*." The list of *essential* and *indispensable* baby items was enormous (even though we would be gone just three months). It seemed we would need to ship everything from bottles, to diapers, clothes, a pack 'n play, a crib, a rocking chair, furniture, and my favorite, an electric baby wipes warmer, to Spain in advance of our arrival.

I would joke that I had heard from good sources that people had been having babies in Europe for quite a while and that I was sure that whatever we actually "needed" we could get there. My attempts to use humor made no difference; some even suggested that we would need a container to ship all the "baby stuff." It seemed that anything less clearly amounted to child neglect and served as further evidence that we had no idea what we were about to do. Like I said before, Kasey took the very different approach of waiting to tell anyone until our trip was imminent and she ended up doing much better. It was, however, an eye-opening experience for me to have these interactions with so many people. The experience taught me that sometimes it is best to keep certain decisions private even if only for a little while. My overly concerned friends (that did not know Kasey very well) concluded that I was about to do something horrible to my poor complacent wife and innocent newborn. In their view, this was clearly my doing and, like Don Quixote dragging Sancho Panza all over Spain in his misguided adventures, Kasey had to be blinded to my madness and we would surely both regret it.

A Note on Nesting

*"Wealth consists not in having great possessions,
but in having few wants."* — *Epictetus*

Many parenting websites will suggest that the months before the birth of a child are a time for "nesting" and further, that this is a natural instinct (which rather suspiciously requires you to purchase lots and lots of stuff from sponsors of the website). Magazines bombard you with lists of "necessary" items which your mother and grandmother, although they may be quick to get onboard at the baby shower, will probably tell you they never used or needed. And any mother-to-be who has ever entered a baby store to start a registry will no doubt recall the overwhelming number of must-haves and, I dare say, most will appreciate the pressure the typical young mother is under to conform to certain expectations (which all too often are manufactured by the multi-zillion dollar baby industry). Baby super stores even offer the services of registry specialists who will eagerly dedicate all day to making sure you do not miss anything.

While I must confess here that I am not personally crazy about shopping and may be described by some as a bit of a minimalist, I am no scrooge. I am not suggesting that there is no place for a baby shower to celebrate the joy of the upcoming birth or to help defray the true costs associated with the new child. We did, in fact, enjoy more than one shower and I am grateful to those people in our lives who wanted to celebrate with us by hosting one. I have also been a participant in many showers for friends and family, including what they call in The South, a "pounding," where a young bride gets a pound of flour, a pound of sugar, a pound of detergent and so forth to stock her pantry. But in keeping with the theme of this book—leading a more deliberate life—I do believe that we should each examine for ourselves what we really need and want. For far too many, it seems those decisions are dictated by the motives of advertisers or social pressures. This is true particularly as we begin a family, a time which seems rivaled only by wedding planning, as the prime time to become a marketing target. After all, when it comes to our children, we all want the best and may fear that "more is better" or "better safe than sorry." This is, no doubt, a marketer's dream. But for us, the decision to dramatically reduce the amount of "stuff" associated with welcoming our daughter into the world meant that we were not weighed down and could easily travel abroad. In hindsight, I certainly would not have traded this experience for more "convenience," and, the truth is, we never missed a thing!

Money Talks

"In polite society, one should never discuss politics, religion or money." — Unknown

Something I find amazing to this day is that *nobody*, not even once, asked us how much the trip would cost or how we could afford it. I have heard many times people talk about the $10,000 they would need for just a one week trip to anywhere in Europe. Considering that so many people think that a European vacation is so expensive, I can't imagine how much they estimated our three month trip (including having a baby) would cost or how they thought we would pay for it.

I don't know if people never thought about it, but having been asked even the craziest questions, I still find it hard to believe that no one wondered. Even the people that tried their best to talk us out of it never suggested that the expenses of such a long trip would be too high for a couple about to have their first baby. I wonder if money is still such a taboo topic that no one dared to ask. I assure you, aside from the health of

Kasey and the baby, affordability was my number one concern all along.

A personal goal of mine was to keep the whole trip as inexpensive as possible. Besides the obvious reason, I wanted to prove to ourselves my theory that it was possible to live in Europe for at least the same amount of money that it cost us to live in Florida, if not less. Based on previous trips and by looking at property rentals and other expenses online, I estimated that being in Barcelona for three months would cost us about the same as staying in our condo in Florida plus the airfare.

If we rented out our home while being away, we could not only breakeven, but even make some money (Kasey would not let me do that, though, because she did not want any surprises when we got back with our new baby). Our biggest expense was the apartment rental in Barcelona. In order to accommodate Kasey's requirements, it needed to be by the beach, which was a highly desirable area in the summer. Since we were only renting for three months, and during peak season, we paid a premium. Still, it cost us about the same as our mortgage payment plus utilities in Florida, although we could have gotten a bigger apartment in another good location (not by the beach) for half the price. Our second biggest expense was the airfare, which cost about $2,200 for both of us round trip, plus an additional $120 for our daughter on the way back. Food and entertainment were about half of what it cost us in South Florida. With me working from home and Kasey taking the subway to school, we did not spend money on gas except when renting a car for weekend trips (we both had long commutes in the U.S. so this was a real savings for us). Since I was home all day and Kasey came back from school around 2:00 p.m., I cooked a lot more and we did not eat out as much as we did in Florida.

We also had some unexpected savings. Since our cars were parked in a garage for three months, we received a deep discount on our car insurance and we discontinued our cable and Internet service while we were away. Also, since we knew that carrying anything back on the plane would be a hassle, we hardly did any shopping while in Spain. With so much to see and explore in a city like Barcelona, most of which was free, going to a mall was the last thing on our minds.

I regularly keep decent records of how we spend our money and, during our trip, I was even more careful tracking our expenses. Including those medical expenses not covered by our insurance, Kasey's Spanish classes, restaurant meals, car rentals and the hotels we stayed in on our road trips, the final tally showed that we spent a little less than we had in the previous three months in our routine Florida life. Had Kasey agreed to rent our condo in Florida while we were away, we would have actually come out ahead.

I think Kasey would have been elated with the experience even if it had cost us a chunk of money, but knowing that we had pulled it off on the cheap was a particular success for me because I wanted to make sure that we could repeat this experience. Since I had my sights set on an even longer stay in the future, breaking the bank on this trip would have made it that much more difficult for us to repeat this feat, not to mention that with a new baby we needed to be responsible with our finances now more than ever.

Preparations

Ducks in a Row

"We're surrounded by people who are busy getting their ducks in a row, waiting for just the right moment. . . . Getting your ducks in a row is a fine thing to do. But deciding what you are going to do with that duck is a far more important issue."
— Seth Godin, blog post "Whatcha Gonna Do with That Duck?"

I must pause here to applaud my extraordinary husband for all the time, effort and careful consideration he put into making this dream a reality. In particular, he lovingly dedicated himself to researching Barcelona to find an incredible place for us to live. Apparently, I am a little high maintenance in this regard. I really wanted to be conveniently located to everything, and beachside, all without spending a fortune. I will let Erick elaborate on his challenges, but here are the things I needed to figure out.

First, I was pregnant. How long could I fly? Would They let me? I began by researching airline policies for pregnant flyers. Each airline is different so if you are thinking this adventure sounds like a great idea, it is important to check. Some claim to prohibit travel after a certain point, while others require a doctor's note if you are close to your due date. The general consensus, though, is that it is reasonable to fly up until about 35-36 weeks. To be clear, flying itself poses no actual risk of harm to mother or child, except for maybe an increased risk of blood clots from sitting too long (as mentioned in the introduction, I wore compression stockings, which can help avoid this problem) or severe turbulence (a risk I determined was lower on an airplane than during my daily commute to and from downtown Miami on I-95).

The only real worry then is that you might go into labor at a very inconvenient time. Although I was not high-risk for premature delivery, I did not want to test this. After all, it would be me laboring at 40,000 feet. In fact, just weeks before we left, a woman gave birth aboard a plane headed for Miami and my coworkers could not resist forwarding me the article. But despite the potential perks for our daughter had she been born *en route* (airlines have been known to give free tickets for life to "mile-high" babies), we decided to travel about five weeks before she was due.

I chose an airline that did not have any stated policy restricting pregnant travel. Nonetheless, I will admit that I did try on different outfits prior to our departure to see which one made me look "less" pregnant. In reality, there was no disguising my enormous belly and everyone was more than gracious to us during our travels. Also, to minimize any potential hassle, and just in case They asked, I did have my doctor sign a note stating my due date. It was never requested by anyone. My employer worked with me to schedule my maternity leave around our travel plans. I still took the same amount of time off (four months per the employer's policy), but I moved it up a bit.

For peace of mind, I also wanted to know that I would have a doctor waiting for me in Spain should I need one right away. How much would that cost? And how do you find a doctor in another country? This turned out to be remarkably simple. I searched my insurer's website just like I would have in Florida. I entered: Barcelona, OB/GYN. A female doctor popped up and she even spoke English! In the age of the Internet, it is easier than ever to get all the relevant information about someone's credentials and I was impressed. I actually found more information about my doctor in Spain than my treating OB/GYN in the U.S. I called from Florida and scheduled an appointment for the day after we would arrive. I had a truly wonderful healthcare experience while we were away, but more on that later. As it turned out, my insurance had international coverage and we did not pay any more in Spain than we would have in the U.S. Since my doctor was listed on the insurer's website, she was even treated as an in-network provider. This was one more stumbling block overcome!

Logistics: In a Nutshell

"Adventure is just bad planning." — *Roald Amundsen*

Some matters did pose questions that needed to be answered and we were very diligent in our research. Kasey and I confirmed, independently, and prior to our departure, most of the information below. It was important for us to make sure that neither of us had misunderstood something and that we were not making any incorrect assumptions. Most of the items below would have needed to be addressed regardless of where our baby would be born and/or in advance of any extended trip and we simply tailored our research to our specific plans.

Airlines: We researched airlines online and confirmed that, up to a point, most don't care if you travel pregnant. Some had recommendations about not flying in the last few weeks, while others required a doctor's note saying that it was safe to fly. We chose Delta Airlines since they had the most direct flights and had no restrictions whatsoever.

Apartment Rentals: I looked for apartment rentals online and found several Barcelona based websites oriented toward long-term rentals for tourists. They had pictures and information in English and condos all over the city. The rents were about the same as in South Florida and one could make the reservation online with a credit card or call them directly and make a wire transfer. Like in the U.S., prices vary a lot depending on location, amenities and length of stay.

Banking and Currency: We had direct deposit with our employers and already received and paid all of our bills online. Getting euros is something that one can do with a debit card in any ATM machine in Europe the same way you would get cash in the U.S. Visa and MasterCard are also widely accepted throughout Europe. Prior to our departure, I also purchased some euros in our local bank branch to take with us just in case we had a problem with our cards.

Hospitals: We looked up some hospitals available through our insurance and were able to call them directly and get information (even in English). It turns out that it is not uncommon for British citizens to go to Spain for medical services, especially if it requires hospitalization. (Better to recover by the Spanish Mediterranean Sea than in England's weather I guess.)

Insurance: We called our insurance company (Blue Cross) and they confirmed that they would cover the birth expenses overseas in pretty much the same way as if we were in the U.S. They even had a list of in-network doctors and hospitals in a large number of countries. We looked for Barcelona and found a number of clinics, hospitals and doctors that we could contact prior to our arrival. There were several that had English speaking doctors and staff. The only difference was that we had to front the costs and then submit claims forms to be reimbursed later.

Maternity Leave: We confirmed that both Kasey and I were entitled to take up to 90 days of unpaid leave when having a baby. Many employers are flexible and have different options, but this is the minimum required by U.S. federal law for companies of a certain size.

Medical Concerns: We researched whether there were any medical risks related to flying pregnant and found none. A plane would obviously be a very inconvenient place to be if Kasey happened to go into labor early so we made sure with the doctor that Kasey was not at risk for premature delivery. To be extra careful, we flew a full five weeks prior to Kasey's actual due date and all our plans were contingent on Kasey having a healthy and uneventful pregnancy. Kasey requested her medical records from her U.S. doctor before we left and gave them to her doctor in Spain.

Nationality: Like most other nationalities, the American citizenship of the parents is always inherited by the children, no matter where they are born. All we needed to do for our child to get an American birth certificate and passport was go to the American Consulate in Barcelona and present her Spanish birth record along with our American passports. Unlike every country in North and South America, however, being born in Spain does not automatically entitle a person to Spanish citizenship.

Our Home: We lived in a condo and all we needed to do to go anywhere was lock the door on the way out. One can also request that the post office hold one's mail for period of time or forward the mail to a friend or family member's address.

Visa Requirements: Different countries have different visa requirements when it comes to travel in Europe. U.S. citizens can visit Spain for up to 90 days (within a 6 month period) as tourists without obtaining a visa. We did not need any paperwork other than our passports because we stayed just under 90 days. This was super convenient for us as it was just the right amount of time for maternity leave!

Work: Kasey was getting 16 weeks of unpaid maternity leave, and I was planning to request 90 days of unpaid family leave, and if my employer agreed, I would continue to work remotely.

What About My Job?

"When your values are clear to you,
making decisions becomes easier." — Roy E. Disney

This would be the last piece in the puzzle. I knew that, by law, I was entitled to take up to 90 days of unpaid family leave if caring for a sick relative, or if having a baby. This is normally called maternity leave (because mothers must take time off after having a baby). Many professional women in the U.S. don't even take off the whole three months, though, and it is almost unheard of for a man to take this time off. Most men only take a few days and go back to work as soon as possible. I can only speculate about their reasons, but I would assume that the fact that the leave is *unpaid* probably has a lot to do with it. The prevalent idea that women are supposed to instinctively know how to care for a new baby, or that men are useless in these matters, can't help either. Whatever the case may be, I was determined to be there with my wife and newborn from day one, and for as long as possible.

The idea of asking for 90 days off was not appealing to me. I feared that my boss/employer would be so unfamiliar with the concept of "paternity leave" that they would deny my request on the spot. If I pushed the issue by invoking the law, I also worried that I might face retaliation or even get fired before or after our trip.

We decided that I would talk with my employer only after everything was in place and we were as certain as possible that we were actually going. The key factors were making sure that Kasey had a healthy pregnancy and that she could fly without risk. We could only make this final determination within the last two months before our scheduled departure.

Since we had decided to pursue our dream, I had gone over in my head every possible scenario of how the conversation with my employer could go. If my worst fears materialized, I would have to make a decision between fulfilling our dream or, perhaps, losing my job just as we were about to have our first baby. I had many sleepless nights pondering this. I shared very little of my worry with Kasey since I didn't want to stress her, but I kept running different scenarios about how much money we would need to have in savings if I lost my job, and how long it would take me to get another job.

As the week when we had decided it was most prudent to talk with my employer arrived, my stress level got to its worst. One night, I finally shared all my anxieties with Kasey. We talked about the actual risk of losing my job. Since our monthly expenses were pretty low, between Kasey's job and our savings, we would be okay even in the unlikely scenario that I could not find a job for a whole year. We had addressed this possibility many times before and Kasey was surprised that I was still worrying about this so late into our plans.

I realized that my anxiety could not be just about my job or even money. I had to be afraid of something else. Once we started talking, I started searching for my real fears, those we hardly ever acknowledge to ourselves and certainly never talk about with anyone else (because it's embarrassing maybe).

I decided to get it all out and tell Kasey, and, as it turned out, I was also afraid of the mighty They! I was not afraid that They would somehow stop us, but instead, I was afraid of what They would say or even think. Who were They for me? They were Kasey's family, my family and, to a lesser extent, even our friends. As we went through this pseudo psychoanalysis, I finally admitted out loud that my real fear was that since the blame for our "crazy" idea had already fallen squarely on me, if I also lost my job over it, I would be judged as a completely irresponsible husband and father. No matter how great everything eventually turned out, once that judgment was out, I would not be able to change it.

In light of this personal revelation, Kasey was very patient and understanding with me. However, she told me that it wasn't like me to worry about other people's opinions. I further confessed to her (and there always seems to be more to confess once we start digging into our secret thoughts and feelings) that in my heart of hearts, after so much criticism of our plans by almost everyone I knew, I was beginning to think that if I lost my job over this, maybe judging me as irresponsible would be right. Maybe even we would end up concluding that I was the fool that had dragged my trusting wife into something we would eventually regret.

She reassured me that she would never think I dragged her into anything, that this was a well thought out plan, that it was something she wanted to do for herself and that she didn't care if her family judged me and neither should I. She reminded me that I was not inclined to let others sway me and that now was our best opportunity to pursue this dream, and if we missed it now, we wouldn't dare to do it later.

I felt relieved after this conversation and was again amazed at my wife and grateful to God for having married her. I decided to talk to my boss the next day, hoping for the best, but ready for the worst. I should mention that, at the time, I worked in a technology company that translated websites into many languages and two thirds of the staff were foreign born. So, the whole idea, perhaps, would not be received as farfetched as in another type of company.

When I talked to my boss, I explained how important it was for us to teach Spanish to our children, how Kasey's learning was instrumental to achieving that goal and since there would be no other time when we could take three months off to go study the language overseas, this was our opportunity. I had a lot of work that would be hard to hand off to someone else, so I offered to work remotely as well if they preferred (I explained in detail how this could be accomplished). My boss didn't look nearly as surprised as I expected. He told me right away that he didn't see a problem with it, but that he would need approval from upper management. He did say, however, that it was crazy for Kasey to have this baby overseas.

Two days went by and I still didn't have an answer. I was eager to buy the airplane tickets, but I still wanted to know my job situation before deciding on the final dates. I started thinking that maybe I had not explained myself clearly enough when I talked to my boss. I went to him again and submitted my formal time-off request for family leave in writing and clarified that I was only waiting to know if I would be allowed to work remotely.

A couple of days after buying the tickets, I got word that I would be allowed to work remotely as long as my productivity was not diminished. I was asked to sign some documents stating that if there were any problems with my performance while I was away, I would be placed on unpaid family leave, and clarifying that I would be covering all of my living expenses. I was also asked to write in detail how all my functions and responsibilities would be fulfilled while being away. I had done my technology research and was ready for this and happy to sign the commitment documents.

I would be working overseas for three months. This was a surprisingly bittersweet development. Bitter, because I would not be able to travel as much or study French like I wanted. Sweet, because I would keep my job, not lose three months of income and would have the opportunity to maintain my good standing at work.

Courage and *Kairos*

"It is in your moments of decision that your destiny is shaped."
— Anthony Robbins

Courageous was a word often used by our few encouraging friends to describe Kasey before we left (I only remember being called less flattering things), but it was overwhelmingly used by almost everyone to describe Kasey and our experience after we came back. To me, courage was a very interesting word to use in this context since it implied conquering some big fear. I thought that executing our plan would take some ingenuity, creativity, planning, perseverance and maybe some luck, but I never thought that courage would be necessary to have a baby away from "home" and to spend maternity leave abroad. For many people, leaving familiar surroundings and being out of one's comfort zone takes a lot of courage, especially if they are about to have a baby. In our case, we had no family nearby, nor did we feel that we needed additional support other than each other. For us, being away simply meant seeing and learning new things. We found the anticipation exhilarating and looked forward to it. We saw the whole trip as an awesome and very suitable treat as we embarked on the very exciting adventure of starting a family.

Nevertheless, I had my fears. In addition to those that I think most fathers-to-be must experience, I had some other fears related to the trip that needed to be conquered. I was afraid that Kasey would change her mind at any moment. I was afraid that she would have some kind of health complication that would prevent us from going. I was afraid of missing something that would make our plan fall apart at the last minute. I was afraid of losing my job if working remotely didn't work out. But, by far, the biggest fear I had was the fear of missing out on our *kairos* moment. The ancient Greeks had two words for time, *chronos* and *kairos*. While the former refers to chronological or sequential time, the latter signifies the right, opportune or supreme moment; a moment of indeterminate time in which something special happens.

In the 1998 movie *Sliding Doors* we get to see in parallel how the love life and career of the protagonist take very different directions based on whether she catches or misses a subway train. I would like to think that *kairos* moments are not quite so random, but that they are best represented in important decisions that we make in life, although we are seldom aware of the extent of their ramifications. Too often we make these decisions without appreciating how important they will be to our future. Only in retrospect do we realize the full impact they had in our lives' trajectories: lighting up that first cigarette or just saying no; ending that relationship when one first knew it wasn't going to end well or deciding to stay in it way too long; getting behind the wheel that night after having had too much to drink or staying put; staying at one's comfortable secure job or taking the risk and changing careers; taking the normal reasonable path or daring to make that trip that would change one's life.

Kasey and I talked often about the *kairos* moments in our lives. Once we knew that our dream to spend maternity leave abroad was possible, other than a health complication during the pregnancy, we would have no good excuse not to go. We felt that if we did not dare to take this step to reach this dream we would set a terrible precedent and forgo others as well. I don't think that any real courage was displayed on my part to actually go abroad. What actually took courage was pursuing our dream even in the face of so much criticism. With regard to Kasey, I do think that the actual act of being pregnant for nine months and finally giving birth to a human being does takes an immense amount of courage from any woman (no matter where or how she does it). For Kasey to dare to add more uncertainty to this event by going to a foreign country was truly remarkable, especially for a new mom. Seeing her pregnant and being with her during the delivery was the most humbling experience I have ever had or can imagine to this day.

Relative Distance

"Time is relative." — *Albert Einstein*

I had the very ambitious goal of remaining in contact while in Europe without anyone having to make *any* changes in how they reached us. I had two main groups of people in mind: work related people (coworkers/clients) and Kasey's family.

I already had remote access to my office computer in Florida and all I needed was a PC and broadband Internet access in Spain. However, a lot of my work was performed over the phone with clients and coworkers and I needed a solution for that. I started by looking into different available phone plans. I contacted our cell phone carrier and their fees for international roaming were very expensive. I could not expect people who needed to reach us to have to pay long distance so I started searching for an alternative on the Internet. It wasn't easy to find one right away since I didn't know exactly what I was looking for. I knew that one could use the Internet to talk with people anywhere using services like MS Messenger and Skype, but these needed to be installed on the computers on each end of the call and the computers would both need Internet access. (Of course these options are always changing and there are more and easier methods out every day.) Installing and using these services would have been an inconvenience for my coworkers and clients, not to mention that it would have required a certain level of IT knowledge that I could not expect from Kasey's Mom. So, I started asking friends that had family overseas or traveled frequently how they stayed in touch.

One of my friends recommended Vonage. The system seemed to do what I needed and it would cost only $25 a month. This solution was ideal since I could just take a small modem to Europe and be able to receive calls from people that were only using their phones to call a local Florida number (one can get a local number from anywhere in the world) without anyone paying long distance or even knowing where I was. This was pretty good, but it still required me to give a new number to everybody. This was particularly undesirable with my many clients since it would likely lead to me having to tell them that I would be working overseas, and the idea that I would be managing their accounts from a different continent could make them uncomfortable. After several days of wondering how to overcome this last issue, I realized that I could forward our cell phones as well as my office number and private office extension to the new Vonage number. Anyone who wanted to reach us could use the same method they were used to and be rerouted to us in Spain without us having to tell anyone to make any changes on their end. I immediately placed the order to test it. I received a modem in the mail, installed it on my PC, hooked it up to a regular phone and was able to get a local Florida number right away.

Like in most companies today, I had a lot of meetings every week. I agreed with my boss to join all of my office meetings via phone. I would work during the company's normal business hours from 8:00 a.m. to 5:00 p.m. Florida time, which meant that I would be working from 2:00 p.m. to 11:00 p.m. Barcelona time.

For those few that knew that I was going to Europe, it was hard to believe that they could really reach me at the same number. Friends and family were still hesitant to call us thinking that somebody would somehow end up paying an exorbitant long distance fee. In contrast, people that didn't know I was away, continued to reach me at the same numbers they were used to without any concerns.

I was also concerned that Kasey's parents would feel that they were missing their only daughter's first baby's actual delivery because we were in Europe. Even though they would have also missed it in Florida, I still wanted to minimize that sentiment as much as possible. Since Kasey's Mom did not use the Internet, and we could not email her pictures, I was also planning to take pictures and upload them online to a U.S. store where Kasey's Mom could go and pick them up herself. I knew that I could do this, but decided to surprise Kasey's Mom and did not mention it until the pictures were ready.

Lightweight Champions

"There's nothing American tourists like more than the things they can get at home." — Stephen Colbert

Once Erick had found us a home away from home, I had secured a doctor, we had discussed our plans with our employers, our flights were booked, summer school was all lined up and I had broken the news to my family, we just needed to pack! Of all the topics discussed with friends and family, this may have been the most controversial. What *must* one take if you are going to have a baby abroad? Not a question many people had previously considered, but one about which everyone had an opinion. Were we planning to ship strollers, bottles, toys, clothes, a crib or diapers? The short answer was no. Erick and I intended to take only that which we could carry on the plane without paying any extra baggage charges (a goal I am pleased to report we managed successfully both coming and going).

So, on the way to Spain, we had two full-size suitcases we could check, two smaller carry-on suitcases, one small backpack, a diaper bag (that at first doubled as my school bag) and one very pregnant me. Although we could vacuum seal our clothes for maximum space, one realizes very quickly that the real challenge comes at the airport weigh station. Each bag had to come in under 50 pounds, which is actually not a lot.

Being pregnant and intending to lose most of my weight while abroad (as was my hope at least) presented a unique packing challenge for me. We had also discussed traveling to some colder climates so I could not just take my summer best. And, of course, what should we take for our daughter? Fortunately, her teeny-tiny outfits (the same ones that would later look too adorable hanging off our balcony drying in the sun) did not require much packing prowess.

But what about all the necessary baby gear? We seriously considered taking a stroller and, at one point, I thought perhaps we should take the pack 'n play, which we already had, to serve as our daughter's first crib, but ultimately, we decided that it really wasn't practical to take any of those things and that we would just acquire whatever we would need once we arrived. In retrospect, I think this was absolutely the best decision. Of course, we had no trouble finding everything we needed in Barcelona and the only major purchase that we were not able to bring home was a baby swing, which we decided was well worth the money we spent on it (lucky for us, some friends lent us theirs once we returned).

In consulting with friends regarding this issue, my favorite advice came from a coworker who is a mother of two adorable children herself. She said that we should buy everything in Spain so that we would be able to get all the cool European stuff that nobody else had. As it turns out, this was great counsel. The stroller we bought in Barcelona is not available in the U.S. (at least I have never seen it). It was great for us because unlike the car seat/stroller combos we had considered buying, this car seat would lay completely flat across the back seat. So during our lengthy weekend road trips, our daughter was able to rest comfortably in her cozy bassinet-style seat. It also served as an on-the-go portable changing table and newborn crib. And, more than one woman approached me in the mall after our return to ask where we got it. The husband of an old high school friend, who we ran into with her newborn, even commented on our daughter's "pimp ride." Over two years later, we are still strolling.

In order to be able to work remotely and stay in contact without disrupting anyone, I needed a few technological gizmos. Sometimes electronics can be up to 20 percent more expensive in Europe. Therefore, I purchased everything that I would need in the U.S. In my office, I was working with two regular size monitors and I didn't think that I could work effectively with just the little screen on my laptop. Instead, I purchased a new 22 inch monitor that was just large enough to show two screens simultaneously. I also bought the fastest and smallest desktop I could find (the trip gave me a great excuse to get a new PC). I took a regular corded phone to go with the modem for the Internet phone, as well as a GPS navigator, a webcam, a microphone, a personal camera and my cell phone. Packing everything together with the cords, chargers and electricity convertors (from the American 220V to European 110V) took an entire large suitcase that was barely under the airline's weight limit. I only had another small carry-on suitcase to use for my clothes and a backpack where I carried two pairs of shoes.

I must admit that bringing all these electronics turned out to be excessive and unnecessary. The land phone was bulky and needed to be replaced after a couple of weeks. Our cell phones and GPS navigators were not compatible with the European system and did not work. I never used the webcam and the new monitor burned out after just two weeks in Spain. If I had to do it all over again, I would just take a light laptop with a bigger screen, a voice modem and a smart phone (with a GPS) compatible with the European system.

Traveling in the summer meant that the clothes we were taking were smaller and lighter, which was fortunate because we would not have had room for bigger jackets. Neither Kasey nor I would be going to an office every day so we wouldn't need work clothes and the apartment we rented in Barcelona had a washing machine. We hoped to travel within Europe and take lots of pictures and we did not want to have the same outfits in all of them, so we still packed more clothes than we needed. Even though we traveled more than I ever thought possible, I still had a couple of pairs of pants and shirts that I never wore during the whole three months. It may be hard to believe that we traveled so light, but I still think we took way too much.

Somos Campeones

We Actually Did It!

*"In the name of God, stop a moment,
cease your work, look around you."* — Leo Tolstoy

We arrived at the Barcelona International Airport at 9:00 a.m. We had actually done it! It was sunny, hot and humid, and even after a long night and our in-flight adventure, Kasey looked surprisingly fresh and happy. I, on the other hand, was still concerned about the apartment we had rented. Would it actually look like the pictures online? And more importantly for me, would it really have fast Internet access as promised? Would all the phones work like I expected? Would I really be able to work remotely? I had foolishly decided not to be happy about anything until I could confirm that.

I wanted to take the train that goes from the airport to Barcelona, make the subway connection to our neighborhood and walk to the leasing office (with our luggage). However, my very pregnant wife convinced me otherwise, and we just took a taxi from the airport directly to the leasing office.

Upon arriving at the leasing office around 11:00 a.m., they offered to keep our suitcases until the apartment was ready at 3:00 p.m. A long-term tenant had just moved out that morning and they were sprucing up the place. Kasey was dying to check out the apartment and the beach that was only a couple of blocks away. I was hungry. Kasey was elated and marveling at the fact that we were actually there. I was still worried about installing the computer and testing the phone, but being forced to wait, we walked to the beach to get lunch. I continued to refuse to celebrate with Kasey until I could confirm the functionality of my tech gizmos.

Small World

"Travel is not really about leaving our homes,
but leaving our habits." — Pico Iyer

Seeing our apartment for the first time, I realized that we had indeed entered a small world. It was not exactly what we expected from the photos online. Not that they were necessarily misleading, but in real life, it was *very* small. The entire place was less than 400 square feet and it had some very "eclectic" artwork on the walls, which included several full-color abstract paintings of sultry jazz musicians in the bedroom, and, in the living room, an enormous outline of a female face with bright red lips. By way of comparison, our two bedroom, two bath condo in Florida was about 1,100 square feet (and had somewhat less distinct artwork). Our new place had one *tiny* bathroom. It had a very small shower stall and the front edge of the toilet seat was only a few inches from the wall requiring some serious maneuvering from my very pregnant self to use either. The apartment had a small washing machine in the kitchen, but no dryer. It was, however, equipped with a clothesline which extended out over the street from our balcony. This would be a first for me. Although I had frequented many a laundromat in my college days, I had always had the luxury of a dryer. The Barcelona tour buses that drove through our neighborhood (Barceloneta) gave visitors a view of the beach if they looked toward our place. I have often wondered how many tourists went home with a souvenir photo of our underwear! Having said that, though, it felt just like we were living in a postcard.

The apartment was also on the fourth floor—with no elevator. We were under the impression from the website that we had rented a second floor apartment (we didn't know the building had a mezzanine floor and a flight of stairs leading up to the first apartment). And it was not just a matter of climbing the stairs each day, but bringing up groceries, luggage, the stroller and our daughter. I was also concerned that I might struggle with the stairs in my final pregnant weeks and after the delivery. As it turns out, I had no problems and, in fact, credit the stairs in part for my quickly getting back into shape. To make it more interesting, when we arrived, the A/C was broken and it was about 95 degrees outside. Aside from me being one hot pregnant lady, if there is anything that can make Erick grumpy, it is being hot or hungry. (I have since learned to bring along snack bars for him just in case.) By the time we reached the apartment that day, thankfully we had just eaten lunch and we were able to contact the landlord right away about the A/C. It was repaired within the week and we spent most of those first few days on the road anyway so we didn't suffer it too much. I also really cannot complain, though, because as I later discovered, most of the students in my Spanish classes, some of whom were living in Barcelona long-term, had never had A/C because of the expense (or an elevator for that matter). Needless to say, I didn't get much sympathy when I rather naively shared a story about my "hardships" in class.

Don't get me wrong though, the apartment was not all bad. As they say in real estate, what matters is location, location, location! As requested, Erick had found us a place just a minute's walk from the beach boardwalk and our balcony had a side street view of the Mediterranean. We were only a ten minute walk from the subway and all sorts of restaurants, parks and attractions in the old Gothic part of town. And, by the time we left, I had become very attached to our cozy apartment. It was the place where we brought "home" our first child and became a place that I will forever hold a tender spot for in my heart—weird artwork and all!

Mission Accomplished

"Eighty percent of success is showing up." — Woody Allen

As soon as we were able to get into the apartment, I set about testing the computer and the phones. After an hour unpacking and installing everything, I called a friend using the Internet phone and asked him to call my Florida mobile and office numbers. All the calls were properly forwarded to our place in Barcelona. I was able to get online and connect to my office!

I had confirmed that I could talk to anyone in the U.S. without having to pay long distance charges. People from anywhere could reach us dialing our same old Florida numbers. Working remotely was now a reality for me. And, if the phone and email were not enough, through Facebook we were able to keep in touch with many people the same way we would have had we stayed in Florida.

The apartment was even smaller than we expected, but Kasey liked it and she was as happy as a person could be. She called her parents to let them know we had arrived and that she was feeling well. All my tasks were accomplished! I was now ready to relax and begin enjoying being in Europe.

For Kasey's parents, the sense that we had gone really far away started to dissipate after a few weeks. They eventually got used to the idea that they could call their daughter whenever they wanted without paying long distance fees. Since we were six hours ahead, Kasey's Mom was getting printed pictures in her local Walgreens on the same day we had taken them. I cannot stress enough how big this was for Kasey's Mom; she *loves* pictures. Every time we called to tell her that a new set was ready, she would get very excited and run to get them. She repeatedly said that she felt like she was traveling with us (without any of the stress she associates to actual traveling). Since she is not a Facebook user and does not have email access at home, being able to send her pictures she "could touch" was especially great once our daughter was born.

After our daughter arrived, some friends that we don't speak with often and who didn't know that we were in Europe called to congratulate us. Even after talking with them, I couldn't tell for sure if they really believed that we were in Spain. All these things really proved to us that today, more than ever, it is possible to live almost anywhere in world without losing touch or feeling disconnected from anyone as long as one has good Internet access. The world has become a small place indeed.

Neither Here Nor There

"The single biggest problem with communication is the illusion that it has taken place." — George Bernard Shaw

In addition to the two concerns I have already mentioned (heat and hunger), as soon as we landed in Spain, Erick was absolutely preoccupied with an overwhelming *need* to go to France. In contrast, from the moment we arrived, I was just excited to be in Barcelona and could not wait to explore our neighborhood and the larger city. At first, I could not understand Erick's urgency in wanting to immediately rent a car and head over the border. I mean, we had just gotten *here*! I wanted to see what was going on right in front of us. In hindsight, I've realized several things about those first few days. First, Erick loves to work on his language skills and he thought that since he already spoke Spanish there would be nothing for him to learn in Spain. (He has since changed his mind.) Second, he seemed to have the idea that if we were near the beach, we were not *really* in Europe. He would joke (sort of—I think he was fairly serious) that we should "go to Europe" for lunch. By that, he meant that we should go to the Gothic quarter of town that was about a 15 minute walk from our apartment. To him, "Europe" apparently required at least a decent plaza, a really old cathedral and a language foreign to him (and at least at first, a pitcher of sangria). Erick was also concerned that if we did not do some traveling when we first arrived, we may miss the chance. After all, I might become too uncomfortable to travel in the last weeks of my pregnancy (and I didn't want to risk it) and neither of us could predict for certain what might happen after the delivery. He had this vision of himself, like a locked up cat, working at his computer each day and staring out the window at Europe, but unable to go out and explore. Of course, that would make anyone a little depressed. Looking back, it all made sense to me, but at the time I could not appreciate why he seemed discontent upon our arrival.

I can remember us sitting on a park bench the day after we arrived after my first doctor's appointment on Thursday morning. It was clear that Erick had his heart set on going to France that first weekend. The following Monday was the 4th of July work holiday for him, but I was also set to start my Spanish classes. I was not keen on the idea of missing my first day, so after some discussion, we decided that we would head out for the weekend, but be back by late Sunday night. Unlike our later trips, this one was a little ill-advised. We did not make any plans, book any hotels or even really know where we wanted to stop each night. Erick would also later kick himself for not learning even a little French before we left (not even the numbers so we could accurately buy gas).

From the moment we started planning *The Baby Voyage*, I had been lobbying for France—anywhere in France where I could study French and be truly immersed in the European lifestyle. I had, however, acquiesced to spending maternity leave in Spain and was finally able to rent an apartment by the beach like Kasey wanted, although finding it had been quite a challenge. Other than wanting it to be close to the beach, the best Kasey could say when I asked her to give me a criteria for what she wanted was, "I'll know it when I see it." When we arrived in Barcelona I was quite relieved to see Kasey excited about the apartment. However, coming from South Florida, being by the beach, in a neighborhood filled with tourists on vacation and knowing that I would be working for the next three months was a far cry from what I had envisioned for our time in Europe. I thought that the only redeeming aspect about this location was that it was only an hour and a half from France. It was clear to me that we had postponed the French learning experience to a future time. After having had such a hard time finding an apartment online that Kasey liked, I figured that the only way to pick a place in France for our next extended trip would be to go there with her and get her opinion on the spot. Not knowing if we would have an opportunity to go to France after the baby was born, I figured that our first weekend might very well be my only opportunity to get Kasey's feedback on some French towns by the Mediterranean. The following three months would prove my fears completely unfounded and we would have an amazing experience, but at this point with the goal of finding a destination for a future trip on my mind, we rented a car and headed toward the French border just two days after our arrival in Spain.

I had only two goals for our first mini-trip: enjoy the scenery along the French Riviera and not go into labor. I totally missed that Erick had an entirely different agenda. As a result of our lack of communication on this point, this trip resulted in more conflict that we probably encountered during the entire remainder of our time in Spain. At first, the trip seemed to be going well. The first night we easily found a really cool little town with a great hotel where we enjoyed a delicious French dinner. We strolled along the waterside and had quite a romantic evening. This fit my idea of an ideal "babymoon."

The next day Erick began to get a little agitated with me though. He would constantly ask me questions about how I liked this particular place and what specifically did I like about this or that. He seemed annoyed if I did not have a clear answer or if I did not seem fully engaged in the debate. For the most part, we were only seeing small seaside towns—none of which I found particularly appealing for anything more than a one-night stand. Despite my rural upbringing, I have come to realize that at my core, I am a city girl. It had not occurred to me that Erick saw this trip as a fact finding mission (and perhaps the only opportunity we would have) to check out potential future places to live for longer periods. He seemed to be city shopping, whereas I was just sightseeing.

The second night we also ran into trouble finding accommodation. We drove well past a large city and into a quaint small town where we thought we would stay. Unfortunately, after several attempts there was no room at the inn (even for a pregnant lady). By then, it was very late and we had been driving for hours. My feet had begun to swell from the long car ride and I was uncomfortable and cranky. Although we were really struggling with the language barrier in this smaller community, it eventually became clear that due to a festival that day, we would need to drive all the way back to the city we had just come from in search of a room, and there was still no guarantee. I will admit that I had a bit of a meltdown that night, mostly I think from exhaustion. It was the one time I felt as though I had pushed myself past my limit. We did eventually find a hotel in the city and finally got some sleep. The next day, Erick and I had a long conversation about what had been going on between us. We finally understood that we simply had different expectations about this particular adventure. Our next trips went much smoother thanks to a little more planning and a lot more communication.

A Different Time

"Happy the man, and happy he alone, he who can call today his own: he who, secure within, can say,
Tomorrow do thy worst, for I have lived today." — Horace

My work routine was pretty much the same as it had been back at home. A large part of my job was conducted over the phone and I would receive phone calls from clients and coworkers all day while sending emails, attending meetings and working on the computer. Many of my clients and even coworkers in the Florida office that I spoke to on a regular basis never even knew that I wasn't in the same building.

Since I was working on Eastern Standard Time, I didn't actually have to start working until it was 2:00 p.m. in Barcelona. While Kasey went to school every morning, I had plenty of time to sleep in, buy groceries, go to the beach and even cook lunch before Kasey got home. And yet, I still started working remotely before many people had even arrived at the Florida office. During my grocery shopping trips, and within just a few blocks of our apartment, I was able to buy everything we needed, including fresh fruits and vegetables, fresh bread and the delicious Spanish hams and cheeses. I would go on these trips every couple of days and in the process became very familiar with our favorite food vendors in the neighborhood. Sometimes when Kasey would stop for groceries on her way home from school, the ladies that sold us the ham and cheese or the bread would even tell her if I had already bought some earlier that day.

From 2:00 p.m. until 6:00 p.m., I felt as though I was in Florida working in the office. Then, as everybody in the office went out for lunch, I would go with Kasey to the *tapas* bars nearby, often having a jar of sangria that was cheaper than a soda or water. In the U.S., coworkers would have been approaching me to join them for lunch at the same handful of places (and to talk about work). Instead, I was having daily dinner dates with my wife in Europe! In the middle of the summer, the sun did not go down until almost 10:00 p.m., and I worked until 11:00 p.m. Therefore, the rest of the day after lunch went by quickly, and instead of dreading the traffic during my hour-long drive home in the U.S., I was already home and ready to go to bed after a shower, knowing that in the morning, I could sleep in and even go the beach if I felt like it. On my weekends in Florida, I mostly wanted to stay home to rest from the daily two-hour commute during the week and we spent much of our precious leisure time driving around running boring errands. In Barcelona, with my new schedule, I was sleeping in and relaxing every morning. Since I wasn't driving at all during the week, all of a sudden, I had two extra hours every day. When the weekends arrived, I was full of energy and eager to go out, explore the city and even go on road trips.

While my Florida work life had come with me to Barcelona without any hiccups, everything else was drastically different; my commute was gone, my mornings were like lazy weekends, my boring lunch hours were now romantic dates and I was well rested and full of energy for weekends filled with fun and adventure.

Escuela de Verano

"Language is the blood of the soul into which thoughts run and out of which they grow." — Oliver Wendell Holmes

As I noted up front, a huge motivation for going to Spain (Erick obviously wanted France) was for me to work on my Spanish. Since I would not be working, I would be free to spend my days in class. I did not, by the way, have the delusion that I would return from my three months abroad with a newborn baby and fluent, but I hoped it would be just the jump start I needed to see real progress. Both Erick and I began searching for options, and Erick pointed me toward my first language school (I tried two while in Barcelona). I attended my first series of classes through a program at the Autonomous University of Barcelona (UAB). I have always enjoyed the energy of a university setting, but as an added bonus, the language classes here were taught in a building with a storied past.

The *Casa Convalescència* is part of the *Hospital de la Santa Creu i Sant Pau* (this is Catalan—the native language of the region), which was designed by Lluís Domènech i Montaner, a celebrated architect from the early 1900s. He also designed the *Palau de la Música Catalana* in Barcelona among many other sites. With its ornate tile work and vaulted brick ceilings, the structure is a beautiful example of Catalonian Modernism. Originally used to host hospital patients (I was told while studying there that people would better heal in such a beautiful setting) and later for a church, in 1969, the building was converted for use by the university. The hospital complex was named part of UNESCO's Cultural Heritage for Humanity in

1997. Yes, I thought, this would be my introduction to life in Barcelona!

I registered for classes beginning on Monday, July 5th, which was just a few days after we were scheduled to arrive on Wednesday, June 30th. But first, I was required to take an online test to assess my level of proficiency. Although I had studied Spanish for several years in school, it had been a *long* time (more than a decade). Therefore, I must make a confession here. Since I didn't want to start over with *hola*, I may have cheated just a little on the placement test. Even worse, I enlisted Erick to help me. Being the consummate student, I am not proud of my actions. But in my defense, I was confident that I would catch up. And for once, these classes were just for me. There would be no credits and no grades! There was also to be an oral placement exam, but I figured I'd cross that bridge when I came to it.

In my experience, there are basically two types of language learners. There are those who throw themselves headlong into the process talking to every stranger who will listen on the street never concerning themselves with looking foolish or making mistakes. These people are single-minded in their pursuit of speaking the new language and I believe generally do very well. Then are those that diligently go to class, study all the verb tenses and avoid saying a foreign word to anyone until that magic day when they intend to speak with accent-less fluency. They attempt to avoid all the painful mishaps and mispronunciations suffered by the other group. My husband is one of the former (see his experience in Bordeaux as a prime example) while I identify much more with the let's-learn-it-before-we-speak-it crowd. While learning English in Denver, Colorado, Erick tells me he would go through the grocery store line five times in a row to buy his items individually just so he could practice his dialogue. Just when he was ready for the question, "Paper or plastic?" the clerk would change it up and ask, "What kind of bag?" He may have been frustrated, but he learned. For me though, I still wanted the structure of the classroom in addition to practicing on the street.

So, the morning after we arrived back from our first trip to France, I backed my diaper bag/book bag and headed off to *escuela de verano* (summer school)! I was unsure of what to expect and actually found myself filled with first day jitters. I guess it was, in part, just the idea of "going back to school." But in hindsight, I also put way too much pressure on myself to "succeed" at learning Spanish while in Spain. I didn't exactly think that I could achieve fluency in three months, but I was nervous that I would somehow waste the opportunity. And although Erick was not placing any sort of expectation on me, he is quite the language enthusiast and I knew he would have loved the opportunity to learn a new language himself. Since he already spoke Spanish, I felt that this was "my trip" in the sense that he would have chosen a different country. As a result, I gave myself way to hard a time about the whole thing.

But that morning, walking down our four flights of stairs and across Barceloneta to the metro stop, I was also just savoring the experience of city living. I had never really lived in a proper city (Miami doesn't count) and riding the subway for me was still a novelty. And, as an added bonus, since I was way-pregnant, I always got a seat. I rode the 15 minutes to my stop near the UAB language school and climbed the stairs to the surface. I thought I should take all the stairs I could since I still had more than four weeks to go before my due date and was worried that I would begin to struggle with the stairs at home. I arrived at the school (which was beautiful) and registered for my oral placement exam. I was unreasonably nervous about this. A very friendly director then came in to chat with me and assess my level. He asked, *¿de dónde eres?* (where are you from). I did not understand and sat there looking confused. After a few more pretty basic questions, he commented that it was weird that my oral proficiency was so low given my online test. (Hmmm.) He also told me to relax. I think he thought I might go into labor. He determined that I should be put in a low level intermediate class and escorted me to a room almost exclusively filled with college-age students ready to be divided into their respective groups. He also made one of them get up and give me a seat. With the exception of one instructor, I was clearly the most pregnant person in summer school. (Some of the younger students even looked at me like I was a scandal for getting pregnant while I was still in school!) And guess what? My class was on the fourth floor. Stairs—here I come.

Because of my approaching due date, I attended school at UAB for only three weeks, but most of the students were on a four week program and many were getting credit from their home universities. We would attend class four hours a day taught 100 percent in Spanish. Between the classes at UAB and those I took later in my stay, I met students from at least the U.S., England, China, Turkey, Italy, Switzerland, Sweden, Morocco, Croatia, France and Russia. Many of these students were learning Spanish as a third or fourth language and almost all had at least a working knowledge of English. It was certainly the language of chit-chat in the hallways. I had never felt so monolingual!

The second school I attended (beginning several weeks after our daughter was born), Pylmon, was not university affiliated and ran week-long programs for an eclectic mix of students. At this school, they had a two hour grammar class in the morning and then a two hour conversation class in the afternoon. That way you could go to different levels for each. Here, I was pleasantly surprised by the number of tourists that were choosing to do a few hours of language study as a part of their vacation. It would not have occurred to me before this experience, but it is certainly something I'll consider in the future wherever I go. They would come and spend a part of their day in class and then hit the town. Since this school and many others offer culture classes and free group excursions to museums and even night clubs as a way to mingle and have a local show you around, I think it is a great way to get an introduction to a new city. Of the most interesting students I met at this second school, were two sisters only 14 and 15 years old from Croatia. They were in Spain for a few weeks and their parents would drop them off in the morning to work on their Spanish before rejoining them later in the day. I was recruited by the younger sister to be interviewed for her video club project regarding a book they were studying. She managed to get students from all over the world to help her write interview questions in their native language and she then conducted the interview in that language. She even had us all interview in a different spot around campus, presumably to make it appear that she had traveled to the far reaches of the globe for her project.

I genuinely enjoyed my experience at both schools and am thankful to have had the opportunity to take time out from my work to pursue this goal. Although I still have a long way to go, my Spanish proficiency did improve tenfold during our time in Spain and I attribute that in large part to the language schools. Four hours a day of intense focus on an instructor who is speaking and engaging you one-on-one in the new language was, for me, a very helpful exercise. I would certainly do it again.

Of course, I also had ample opportunity to practice my new skills out in the real world. Most people were patient and understanding and generally appreciated that I was making an effort, however flawed. But there was one person in my regular orbit for whom my visits seemed to trigger a panic attack. When the middle-aged pharmacist at the drug store around the corner from our apartment saw me come in, he would start to sweat. Since many items that are kept out on the shelves in the U.S.

are sometimes held behind the counter at the pharmacies in Barcelona, it is more common to require assistance. This man seemed to tremble at the very idea that there may be even slight miscommunication during this interaction. Although I was never seeking anything bizarre or a life-threatening drug, just diapers and the like, I had never seen anyone so nervous! You would have thought he was being tested for his own licensure. But despite his obvious discomfort, he was always helpful, even sometimes to a ridiculous extent. During my favorite encounter, I had successfully requested baby powder, which he had produced, and because as everyone knows, you will be better understood in a foreign language if you SHOUT, he began to loudly read in Spanish the directions from the side of the box, moving his finger under the words so that I could see and read along. As soon as he was satisfied that I understood what I was getting into with my baby powder, and he moved his hand, I saw that the box had the English translation right under the Spanish! I did not point this out and politely thanked him for all his help.

My neighborhood pharmacist is, of course, not alone in his apprehension when it comes to foreign languages. Some people seem to have the irrational fear that anyone speaking a foreign tongue in their presence must be talking about them, while many others seem to simply fear the awkwardness of a social interaction with any person they may not fully understand. Erick had such an experience in France when he went into a store to attempt to purchase gas. He approached the middle-aged cashier and started with his usual French line to elicit patience saying that he did not speak French, but before he could get to his next phrase, she threw her hands to her head and exclaimed in French, "Oh no! That is all I speak!" I guess she had forgotten that it was us that had the problem and not her. After all, we were the ones in need of gas!

If I am honest with myself, though, my greatest underlying worry with regard to speaking in a new language was that I would seem ignorant or completely unsophisticated because I was *so* monolingual. As long as I can remember, I have been a perfectionist and have concerned myself way too much with achievement. My Mom even tells me that when I was just learning to potty train, I peed in my pants once, began to scream and cry inconsolably and then never did it again. So I guess this runs deep. On this trip, I had plenty of opportunities to work on these issues because the simple fact is when you have a newborn baby for the first time, when you are in an unfamiliar environment *and* when you don't speak either local language, humility can be your best friend and ego your worst enemy. One of the most important lessons I learned was that sometimes you just have to admit that you don't have all the answers (since that's pretty obvious anyway) and that everyone needs help.

Despite my perfectionist tendencies, I did manage to discover that there is, in fact, some magic to the "just try" method of speaking a new language. I think the best and most fluid conversation I managed to have occurred on the day I was arguably the most exhausted I had ever been. After our daughter was born, we were of course getting up several times a night for feedings and diaper changes. Erick, to his credit, was 100 percent involved in this endeavor and did try to help me get even more sleep on the nights before I had class. We were both invested in my making the most of this time. But one day in particular, near the end of our stay, I felt as though I had not slept at all. I nonetheless dragged myself out of bed and down to the subway station. During our break from class, I went next door to a small diner and sat at the bar. I ordered a typical Spanish tortilla (a potato and onion omelet) and a Coke. I then actually struck up a conversation with the other patrons having breakfast at the bar and the employees. I think I was so tired that I had lost all my inhibitions about speaking in public. And the crazy thing was that everyone seemed to understand me! Although I may as well have been drunk, I felt like a success. This day was only rivaled by the day after Erick's parents arrived. I was able to go on a stroll down the beach with Erick's father, with our newborn snoozing in my chest carrier, and for the first time have some semblance of a conversation. There were still plenty of hand gestures, but we managed to communicate all by ourselves.

Pickpockets on Shore

"Be careful!" — Mom

Of Mom's voiced worries, only one actually came to pass during our stay abroad. Since we were staying so close to the beach, we were in a fairly touristy part of the city. It was also high season and, as in many cities, there were "professionals" eager and willing to take advantage of the unwary. One day while I was still pregnant, Erick and I went out for a stroll along the beach boardwalk. I was carrying a small purse which I thought I had cleverly secured across my body in order to avoid any "pickpockets on shore." Unfortunately, I had underestimated these guys. After we had been walking for about 30 minutes, I noticed that my purse was unzipped. Despite the fact that Erick had been by my side the entire time, neither of us had noticed when the thief actually managed to get close enough to swipe the wallet from my closed bag. (Later, when we went to the U.S. Consulate to get our daughter's paperwork in order, we met more than one unsuspecting tourist who had managed to lose a passport this way.) Luckily, I had traveled enough to know that it is never a good idea to keep all your credit cards and documents on you while you stroll through a tourist area, but I did lose a credit card, a debit card and some cash. In hindsight, I had no business carrying around that much and resolved to reduce my load in the future. As soon as we returned to our apartment and called the credit card companies to cancel the cards, I also cut the leather tassels from my purse zipper to make it harder to open.

Two things happened as a result of this early incident. First, although we had other credit cards on hand in our apartment, the one we intended to use to front the costs of the delivery had been taken by the pickpocket. Ordinarily this would have been no big deal—just have the credit card company send out a replacement. But we were not at home. We did try to have them send the card to our address in Barcelona via an international courier service, but after several inexplicably failed attempts at finding our place while we were home over a period of a few weeks, we still didn't have the card. Just days before I was due to deliver, we needed to track down the card ourselves. Although we were told that the card was now at the airport distribution center, we could not be sure given the confusion with the delivery service. We decided to make the trek out to the airport to find out.

A cab ride from our apartment to the airport cost about 30 euros each way and would have been about a 30 minute ride. But, if there is one thing Erick cannot stand, it is paying (or over paying) for transportation or parking. I believe that he would drive upward of 40 miles out of his way to avoid a $1.00 toll. (Okay, maybe that's a bit of an exaggeration—but not much.) He also has a sort of childlike fascination with infrastructure and loves exploring "creative" ways to experience as many means of travel as possible. On our honeymoon, I think we tried every conceivable method of transportation except for a donkey—and we only passed that one up because they looked a little too tired that day. For these reasons, Erick did not want to pay for the cab ride when we could *just* take the train. (Did I mention that I was 39 ½ weeks pregnant?) And I had to go on this mini-adventure because only my name was on the credit card. In the end, though, I optimistically and enthusiastically agreed to accompany him to the train station.

We set out just after 11:00 a.m. with every intention of being back at home before 2:00 p.m. when Erick had to start work. By the time we took the subway to the train station, figured out the train schedule and purchased our tickets, it was almost 1:00. Just before the train departed (for a 45 minute ride), Erick ran through the terminal and returned with two tuna sandwiches and a lemonade for us to split. Although we were running late, I think he was still secretly excited about the train ride. Once we arrived at the airport, we began our search for the courier's kiosk. After asking what seemed like a dozen airport personnel without success, and spending almost an hour going in circles, we finally understood that we needed to physically go to the courier's hangar out in the industrial part of the airport. Since passengers don't ever go out there, there was no shuttle or other means to get there other than by foot. We could see a massive commercial park in the distance and off we went. When we were about halfway, I told Erick to go ahead and I'd catch up. The place was going to close at 3:00 and we only had about 10 minutes. "Hurry and just get a foot in the door," I yelled after him, "I'm coming!" Erick arrived just as they were locking up. Apparently having sympathy for me still making my pregnant way along the road, the staff patiently waited. Thankfully, our efforts paid off. With the necessary credit card in hand—we called a cab. I was just hoping that my next scheduled delivery would go a bit smoother.

Minimalist Revelations

"Everything should be made as simple as possible,
but not simpler." — Albert Einstein

The second consequence of our pickpocket encounter resulted in an interesting social experiment for me. I started using cash only for my day-to-day expenses. In my "normal" life, I had become accustomed to always using plastic to pay for even small purchases. Not that this was necessarily a bad idea since we did not have a debt problem and using the card meant that I earned cash back and so on from the credit card company. But many a financial advisor will be quick to suggest that switching to a cash only "diet" will increase your awareness of your spending habits. Although my initial goal was simply to carry less pickpocket bait, an unintended consequence was that I was now much more conscious about what I was buying. Whereas before, I would go to the supermarket for bread and wind up with a bag full of things I realized I "needed" once I got in the store, I found myself in the local grocer with just enough cash to cover what I came in for in the first place. I was also limited by the fact that there was no oversized car trunk to haul my load back home. I would need to carry (or use the stroller's limited capacity to wheel) any purchases back to the apartment and then up the stairs. More than once I found myself either putting something back on the shelf or looking around for a bargain. I did not make nearly as many impulse buys and it felt great.

Although neither Erick nor I is what you would call a "shopper," in the U.S. we still managed to spend a significant amount of our time in big-box chain stores almost every weekend. I would dare say this is true for many American families. Shopping and consumerism have unfortunately become synonymous with leisure time. The concept of a plaza where people come to meet and relax has been replaced by a shopping mall food court. With few exceptions, in our hometown at least, free entertainment is hard to come by and we found ourselves going to a lot of movies and watching way too much television. Even the beaches are lined with private high-rise condos and many public spaces require a fee to park your car.

Having never lived anywhere else, our experience abroad was eye-opening for me. To be clear, I did not set out to radically change my lifestyle or my habits (other than the obvious once our daughter was born). My only goals for the trip were to have a healthy baby girl, improve my Spanish, do some interesting local travel and be able to wear my skinny jeans on the plane back home (which I did by the way—yes!). With the exception of getting to know our daughter, the things I discovered by accident turned out to be in many ways more interesting than the goals I had actually anticipated. Since our return, I have been formally introduced to the concept of minimalist living. I had not really heard this label before we left and, like I said, I did not set out to conduct any particular experiment in this regard, but it happened nonetheless.

First, Erick and I discovered that, in general, we were much pickier about our purchases while on this adventure. In fact, we were almost militant about it. We did not want this experience to end up costing us a fortune and Erick, in particular, was trying to get a realistic picture of how much money it would take for us to live well in another country. We didn't want to spend as if on an extended vacation, and since we were only going to be there for three months, we did not want to purchase anything that would be too cumbersome to take back home. We also simply did not feel the need to shop—even *after* our daughter was born. Since we had so many other activities to fill our time, we did not wind up hanging out in shopping malls and making the type of impulse purchases that had been so common for us.

Particularly with our daughter, had we been back home, I am certain that I would have made many more trips to discount superstores (even if just to get out of the house) to purchase "convenience" items that were simply unnecessary and wasteful. For example, after a week of buying bottled water and hauling it up four flights of stairs, I found myself in serious consultations with Erick over the purchase of a $30 water filter that I am sure I would not have blinked to purchase had we been in Florida. We had revamped the very idea of "necessary" and the crazy thing is we did not feel deprived and we did not miss a thing.

Toward the end of our trip, it also occurred to me that I had not purchased any souvenir to take back with me. As a result, I hastily bought a 5 euro silver bracelet from a street vendor who was selling her wares in Park Güell. In hindsight, I think this purchase was a vestige of an old way of thinking. That is, as though my daughter was not enough, I thought I would need an *object* to remember this time in our lives. I think we are all taught, or maybe have an instinctual urge, to commemorate events with things. What we are really after, of course, is a way to re-experience a certain feeling. Or, I guess in some cases, to be able to prove to ourselves or others that we actually did something. As for me, I realized that I have been unconsciously downsizing my souvenirs for many years. When I was younger, I would buy t-shirts or figurines. And once again, marketers love to sell the idea that we should collect items from different cities (think Hard Rock). Then, as I fancied myself more sophisticated, I started collecting artwork with scenes that showcased a city. Eventually, as I realized that I did not have space for any more pictures on my walls, and that I had married an aspiring photographer, I started acquiring inexpensive pieces of jewelry instead.

Now, though, I am reconsidering the idea of the souvenir altogether. Certainly, if I find something that I really love while we are traveling, and it is easy enough to transport, I still think I might make a place for it in my life. But I do not want to be in the habit of making a purchase simply because I think I *need* to acquire things to help me remember a time or a place. I am therefore now limiting myself to photos and journaling (one thing I wish I had done more of in Europe) to preserve valuable memories. After all, it was the practice of some of the greatest explorers of all time to keep a diary (I can imagine them blogging today). But even if we are not all Charles Darwin exploring the Galapagos Islands, we would do well I think to remember the ways in which our travels change us. A collection of our *thoughts* may be the most valuable treasure we could ever take with us. At any rate, it is probably a better investment than another t-shirt.

Minimalism, I have learned, is about more than just living with less stuff though. It is also about de-cluttering the noise in your life and making way for some mental clarity. So aside from the extraneous stuff and the shopping, another item that disappeared almost without my notice was the television. We had numerous channels available, and many had English programming from the U.S., so this was not the result of a lack of opportunity. When we first arrived, I would occasionally turn on the television to work on my Spanish by watching local shows. We also tuned in to watch the World Cup finals and were certainly amused by the 24-hour coverage of the Spanish soccer team after they won the title. (They actually had live cameras on these guys as they slept on the plane back from South Africa!) I love hoopla and the non-stop parades and commentary were right up my alley. But after that, we simply stopped watching. This was not a decision that we made one day; it just happened. We were just not interested and were too busy enjoying ourselves in other ways. Just before we left, we realized that we had not even turned on the TV in over two months! This was by far the longest I had ever gone without some passive TV watching and I never even thought about it.

People also talk often about "unplugging" as a way to "recharge." In this regard, Erick and I had very different experiences. Erick, by virtue of the fact that he continued working remotely the entire time we were away, stayed pretty well connected to his U.S. life. He spoke daily with his colleagues and clients and worked on his computer at least eight hours a day. He was even operating on East Coast time. This was in itself interesting and a little confusing for me. Not only did we need to be aware of U.S. time, but local time was expressed in "military" time, i.e., 1:00 p.m. is 13:00 and so forth. But other than keeping up with when Erick needed to "go" to work or when he had his "lunch" hour, I did not need to be connected for any reason whatsoever.

By way of background, before we left for Spain, I was a practicing attorney, and although my current job did not require it, I had for many years been immersed in a culture of Blackberries, around-the-clock emails, Outlook calendars and the expectation of immediate client response. Until just one day before we left, I had been involved in litigating some very contentious cases. But once we arrived in Spain, I *completely* unplugged. I barely checked email, I did not really read online news and I only made social calls to friends and family. I did call my office once after our daughter was born (where I had many friends) to let them know we were all well and that I would send pictures. Again, this was not a decision I made ahead of time, but the experience certainly left me with a new perspective on my life and my former habits.

While in Spain, I also began reading the book *Walden*, which I suppose could have started me on my path toward both minimalist thinking and more deliberate living. In brief, the book sets out the musings of the famous author Henry David Thoreau as he experiments with living a "Spartan-like" life in a small hand-built cabin in the woods near Walden Pond, circa 1854. Although in the middle of a bustling city, I related in many ways to his isolation. Because I was removed from daily contact with my "real" life, I felt as if I was on an island of sorts with my small new family, and since I was out of my element in so many ways, I was able to have a sense of introspection about my life that would have been difficult to achieve otherwise. For me, the opportunity to step out of my norm and see with fresh eyes began a transformative process in my life that continues to this day. For this reason, I will forever be grateful for this experience.

Stranger Danger

"As soon as there is life, there is danger."
— *Ralph Waldo Emerson*

Even among all the tourists that visit Barcelona during the summer months, especially in our beachside community of Barceloneta, we still managed to get to know many people in our neighborhood. After just a few weeks, we knew more of our neighbors than we did around our condo building in Florida. We quickly felt as though we had been living there for years. In particular, we became friends with a couple of sweet and very talkative ladies that we would often see walking around in the afternoons. They were especially fond of Kasey because she was pregnant. One of the ladies was almost 70 and her mother was in her 90s. The mother, pleased with her age, would tell us how other than a blister on her foot, the rest of her body was in perfect condition and that she felt as strong as ever. One of the many times we stopped to chat, the older lady complemented me by telling us how much I reminded her of her deceased husband. She was all animated describing how handsome, charming and *simpático* he was, when all of a sudden, as though she remembered something unpleasant, she raised her voice and said that he was also a *pillo*! She made a pause and looked empathetically at Kasey (who was clearly days away from delivering) and with the swiftness of the all the vigor that she claimed to still feel, she smacked me on the face!

I was very familiar with the word *pillo*, and I understood it to mean rascal or mischievous. The old lady meant it also as in a womanizer. Everybody kept talking and smiling as if nothing had happened. It had clearly been a friendly smack and no other forms of aggression seemed imminent. Nevertheless, I was still in shock. The reason for getting smacked was obvious; in my apparent likeness to her husband, I had also reminded her of her of his philandering ways, but that mattered little to me. My main concern at the moment was that a barely five foot tall woman in her 90s had managed to smack me on the face before I could even blink. My confidence in my self-proclaimed ninja reflexes was clearly shaken. When I turned to look at Kasey to share my surprise and utmost indignation, she was laughing!

After kissing the old ladies goodbye (for I am not resentful), I demanded an explanation from Kasey. Why had she just stood there and even *laughed* while she witnessed her husband being attacked by a woman on the street? Chivalry did not allow me to defend myself, but my wife was not bound by such constraints. I told her that I would not accept her pregnancy as an excuse for her impassivity. At almost a full foot taller than the old lady, Kasey could have clearly taken her with only one hand. All that Kasey had to say in her defense in the middle of her laughing was that while she didn't quite understand the whole conversation (that transpired in Spanish), she was sure that I deserved it!

After our daughter was born, we continued to see these ladies during our strolls and they would gush over her while wishing us many more children. While I knew that our baby was in no imminent danger, I'd never again let my guard down near these characters, no matter how adorable and harmless they appeared.

Catalan: A Heavenly Language

"Consequently, you are no longer foreigners and aliens, but fellow citizens with God's people and members of God's household." — Ephesians 2:19

As previously mentioned, Catalan is the native language in Barcelona and although the vast majority of people also speak Spanish (the co-official language), the schooling is conducted exclusively in Catalan and Spanish is only taught as a second language. Street names, public signs and store names are all in Catalan as well. Like Spanish, French, Italian, Romanian and Portuguese, among other European languages, Catalan is a Romance language, meaning that it is a descendant of the ancient Roman Empire official language—Latin. As such, it has similarities with Spanish, but it remains a completely distinct language with its own grammar, spelling and pronunciation, and it is not intelligible to a Spanish speaking person. Catalan is spoken as a native language by around eight million people living in parts of Spain and France and it is the native language of cities as far away as Alghero, Italy.

Kasey and I regularly attended church in Fort Lauderdale and we wanted to continue this important part of our lives while in Barcelona. Picking a church to attend is never easy even in one's own hometown. Selecting a church in another country is a whole different story. I started my search online for a Spanish speaking Protestant church near our neighborhood. Being in a majority Catholic country, and in a city where Catalan is the local language only made my search more challenging. Barcelona, being such an international city, had some churches where the service was given in English to accommodate the large number of expats that live there. However, I was looking for a church where Kasey could continue to be immersed in Spanish and where we could meet more local people. After having to considerably expand the radius of the search, we decided to visit *l'Església Evangèlica Betel* that claimed on their website to have services in Spanish (although suspiciously its name was in Catalan). We decided to give it a try even though it was in a completely different neighborhood, much farther away than we would have preferred. Although this church was even affiliated with the same Presbyterian organization as our church in Fort Lauderdale, it would prove to be a very different experience.

Our first Sunday, we took a taxi to avoid getting lost or being late. I figured that once there, I could get directions to the subway to come home. We arrived just on time for the start of the service. The church was in a very small three story building that did not look like a church at all. There were about 30 people or less in attendance for the service. This was a big contrast to our church in Fort Lauderdale that regularly has around a thousand attendees. Even though their website said that the service was to be conducted in Spanish, most of the attendees were Catalan and would often speak in their language, therefore, about half of the service and many of the hymns were in Catalan. This bilingual service was very interesting for me, but Kasey was not as readily able to tell when they switched languages. She would be excited to see her classes paying off when she understood much of what was said, and then get disheartened when, all of a sudden, she could not understand anything.

The service itself was not that different from what we were used to and we liked the sermon very much. Once the service ended, people started to introduce themselves and welcome us. Everybody was very friendly, but being such a small congregation, where so many were speaking a language that I did not understand, I couldn't help feeling like we were crashing a private event. As we were about to leave, the pastor approached us and invited us to join them upstairs "at the bar."

I respectfully declined, but others insisted that we join them. Kasey was asking me what they were saying. I told her with a smile that I wasn't sure, but that they were talking about something that sounded to me like an invitation to the "bar" upstairs. I told Kasey that clearly they must be using a Catalan word that sounded like "bar" to me, or some kind of local Spanish slang that I did not understand. However, curiosity won the day and everybody seemed so genuine and eager to have us that we decided to stay.

Up the stairs there was a children's room for Sunday school classes and play, and above that there was a big room with an open terrace with several tables and a kitchen. About ten people remaining from the service sat down around a couple of tables on the open terrace and they started serving *tapas* while some of the kids were playing around. They asked me what I wanted to drink: water, soda, wine or beer. A cold beer sounded great in the hot afternoon, but I hesitated to answer, still not sure if I was hearing this right. I had a soda instead. I finally saw a couple of beers arriving at the other table. Later on, after commenting that I had not tried an *Estrella Damm* yet (the local Barcelona brewed beer), they insisted that I have one and I finally acquiesced without feeling uncomfortable.

I should mention that our church in Fort Lauderdale has no objection to responsible drinking, and drinking is normal for most of our church friends. However, I had never imagined a church where beer was served on the premises right after the sermon.

We stayed for about two hours that day, making conversation and enjoying the company and the delicious food. Everybody was very welcoming, but most seemed more comfortable speaking Catalan. Kasey found it extremely amusing that for the first time in her life, people were speaking in Spanish for *her* benefit. I truly enjoy different languages and I was finally having the opportunity to learn some Catalan. I started asking how to say this or that while repeating some words and short phrases that I was beginning to pick up. Pretty soon when speaking with me, they would start speaking Spanish and slowly drift into Catalan (forgetting that I did not speak it). I took advantage of the opportunity to explore with the locals what it was like to grow up and live in a truly bilingual city, where neither language is considered foreign. While many minority languages in Europe are slowly dying out, the Catalan people have made great efforts to keep their language alive. They have made it mandatory in all public schools and institutions, and therefore, all children learn it as first language. They also can't help learning Spanish without much effort by virtue of the fact that they still live in Spain.

Our new friends were very pleased that we had chosen Barcelona as the birth city for our baby and celebrated not only that our daughter would be Catalan, but also that we had properly chosen a Catalan name. They joked that since Catalan would be her "native" language, we would all need to learn it. If that wasn't enough reason for us, they also explained with laughter that everybody knew that Catalan was the language in Heaven. This immediately reminded me of Kasey's Mom's joking concern over future generations in the U.S. speaking a language other than English. She feared that if they did, she would not be able to speak with her descendants in Heaven. I could not wait to hear her thoughts on having to learn Catalan!

As we were leaving that day, I learned that they used the funds raised from these gatherings for the children's programs and that everyone paid for their *tapas* and drinks as if they were in a restaurant. They did not let us pay for anything, however, and the pastor insisted on covering our bill as a welcoming gift. A couple of our new friends even walked us to the metro station and gave us directions on how to get back to our neighborhood.

We felt very fortunate to have had such a great experience with the first church we visited and decided to stop our search. On subsequent visits, we quickly grew very fond of the members of this church and started feeling like we had a church family away from home. We continued to go to *Betel* for the rest of our stay in Barcelona.

The gatherings on the terrace upstairs after the services were routine, and the conversations were always interesting and the atmosphere festive. During our brief time going to this church in Barcelona, I was always pleasantly surprised by the variety of topics of conversation and the diversity of opinions. No one seemed to hesitate in expressing their thoughts, especially when disagreeing. Topics included local and international politics, immigration, interfaith relations, gender roles, history, personal stories, and of course, the very controversial Catalan independence movement. It seemed that no topic was off limits. When there seemed to be a consensus of opinion (such as the importance of speaking Catalan), the conversation quickly moved on to something more interesting where different opinions could be found and discussed. Yet, the tone was always jovial and in good spirits and everyone seemed to enjoy the opportunity to add something unique to the conversation and listen to a different point of view.

I particularly enjoyed the fact that the participants in the conversations ranged from the very young to the very old and included singles and couples, all sharing their different perspectives. This integration is the norm in the culture and was very palpable everywhere we went in Spain. One could always see people of different generations enjoying each other and conversing together.

Later, when our baby was born, taking her to church was a delight. It was like being around family. People gushed over her and made us feel truly cared for, and some even surprised us with gifts for her. When the time to go back to Florida finally came, it was very sad to say goodbye to our new church family. In such a short period of time, we really felt that we had gotten to know these people and when several bitterly complained that they had gotten attached to us, only to see us leave, the fondness they expressed felt very real, and it was mutual.

I don't know what language is spoken in Heaven, but I am sure that our friends at *Betel* have a place reserved for them, and they will likely speak Catalan, even if just for fun.

Clara Catalana

Health Matters

*"Death, taxes and childbirth! There's never any convenient time
for any of them." — Margaret Mitchell, Gone with the Wind*

I was blessed to have a healthy, event-free pregnancy. I was
one of those lucky women who, although a little nauseous
during my first trimester, never really got sick. I did, however,
manage to pack on upwards of 50 pounds before it was all said
and done! I would dread visits to my U.S. doctor because I knew
that the scale would not lie and that I would get another earful
about my weight. Fortunately, I was pretty thin before getting
pregnant and at about 5' 10" I was at least able to spread it out.
Our trip to Spain was also, of course, contingent upon my
having no health complications. So, in addition to the usual
concerns leading up to a due date, I was also anxious that
nothing unusual would happen that would keep us from
traveling. When we were just a few weeks before our planned
departure date, I needed to have a conversation with my U.S.
doctor about my plans and collect my medical records. I was
unduly nervous about this, in part, because so many people had
suggested that this decision was somehow up to my doctor and
that I would need to see if he would "let me go." Although I did
not believe this, and fully intended to make the ultimate
decision about whether to travel based upon the actual facts
related to my health, I still had butterflies in my gut that day.

My U.S. doctor was always kind and, as far as I could tell,
competent, but I had only just begun seeing him after I found
out I was pregnant. It was not as though we had a long-standing
relationship. Our visits consisted of five to ten minute
interactions, but there I was sweating his opinion about this
whole plan presumably because he was an "authority" figure.
As it turned out, I should not have bothered. When I broke the
news, he merely wished me well and immediately agreed to

sign my typed letter that I had brought stating my due date just in case the airline requested one. There was no speech and he offered no opinions. The nurses had plenty more to say—the gist of which was that they wanted to go too!

My healthcare experience in Spain was the best I could have hoped for anywhere. The day after we arrived, Erick and I went to the private hospital where I had an appointment with my doctor. Her office was small and intimate, unlike the busier, more impersonal office of my U.S. doctor. She spoke English, French and Spanish and I enjoyed overhearing her ask a new patient, "In what language will we be speaking today?" On our first visit, Erick and I were invited to sit down in what looked like a study and spent at least 45 minutes discussing our situation directly with the doctor. I have almost never had such an experience in the U.S. and certainly not with my OB/GYN who although polite, always seemed to be under pressure to move on to the patient in the next waiting room. We explained that I was (obviously) expecting to give birth in about five weeks and that we wanted to get an idea of the costs associated with a delivery at the hospital. We knew that our insurer would eventually reimburse us for most of the costs, but we would have some liability and would need to pay the entire amount up front with a credit card. To our amazement, she produced a single page printout which set forth an itemized account of her charges in the event of a normal vaginal delivery and, if necessary, in the event of a C-section. Before we left that day, we were able to have a similar conversation with an administrator regarding any additional costs associated with the hospital and were again provided with a signed one-page quote. By way of contrast, before I left my U.S. doctor's office with my records, I asked the staff to provide me with a breakdown of what I owed them for my visits to date. No one could answer that question. Because of all the insurance red tape, I would need to wait for a bill. I explained that I would be gone for three months and that I could write them a check for what I owed right then, but the cost was seemingly unknowable.

After a visit to a public hospital to comparison shop, which was closer to our apartment, and which was also very nice (more on that later), Erick and I decided to go with our original choice. Over the next few weeks leading up to my due date, I had several office visits and enjoyed seeing a few more ultrasounds of our daughter in utero. The hospital was on the other side of the city from our apartment so, about once a week, I would leave my Spanish class in the early afternoon and take a cab over to the hospital for my appointment. Then I would walk for about half a mile down the hillside from the hospital and take a leisurely bus ride back to Barceloneta where Erick would already be at work. Although my overall health was good, my doctor explained that I did have low levels of fluid. Once she realized how much I had gained, she was also clear that I needed to control my weight (even going so far as to put an "!" beside that point on my records). I guess I couldn't get away from that one! Because of all the walking and the stairs, though, I did stay in decent shape (even losing a few pounds) and felt great right up until my delivery. Just the night before I went to the hospital, I was out walking along the beach with my iPod playing Michael Bublé's "Feeling Good"—*Birds flying high, you know how I feel. Sun in the sky, you know how I feel. Breeze driftin' on by, you know how I feel. It's a new dawn. It's a new day. It's a new life, for me!* Along with our daughter's lullabies, it would become my unofficial *Baby Voyage* theme music.

The week before I was due, the doctor expressed concern that she might need to recommend an induction if my due date passed and my fluid levels did not improve. To make matters somewhat more complicated, I was due on Friday, August 6th and she was scheduled to go on a three week vacation starting Saturday the 7th. (We later learned that the entire country went on vacation for pretty much the entire month of August.

Many restaurants and shops closed completely and posted signs saying they'd be back in a month!) The doctor explained that I could wait until after my due date to see if I would go into labor naturally in the next few days, but that if I didn't by the following Monday, she thought I would need to be induced anyway. There was a doctor on call to assist with her patients in her absence, and she assured me he was excellent, but he did not speak English and I had never met him.

Erick and I had much to discuss. I wanted to deliver with my doctor, who had I come to know and respect, but I was extremely apprehensive about the idea of being induced. I had discussed that I wanted to have as natural a birth as possible. I did not like the idea of unnecessary intervention, especially to jumpstart labor, and was terrified that it would lead to a C-section. When I first learned that I was pregnant, I began paying a lot of attention to the birth stories of friends and family and I was at an age where I knew many women who had recently given birth in a U.S. hospital. I personally knew at least five women who had entered the hospital as low-risk patients, but who nonetheless had an unwanted C-section. I was shocked to learn the actual nationwide statistics. A little Internet research revealed that in 1965, when the rates were first measured, only approximately 4.5% of women experienced a C-section in the U.S. By 2009, that number had jumped to 34% with studies showing Florida (where I would have delivered) as having one of the highest rates in the country. My concerns from anecdotal evidence were clearly not unfounded.

It seemed to me that this change was largely the result of doctors and hospitals using various drugs to "assist" with the labor process and then moving quickly to a C-Section if things didn't progress quickly enough. As I understood it, artificially breaking a woman's water also creates a "deadline" by which the baby must be delivered, making additional intervention more likely. I was not opposed to the use of an epidural, but I had also read that receiving one too early in the process could slow labor and result in an unwanted C-section. It can also be more convenient for doctors and hospitals to schedule a procedure rather than deal with the vagaries of labor, and since more can be charged to the insurance companies for a C-section, it may even be more profitable. Doctors are also faced with an increasingly litigious society in the U.S. so if there is ever any risk whatsoever, no matter how slight, it may be better from their perspective to order the C-section and avoid any chance of a malpractice claim. To me, it seemed there was a lot of upside to a C-section for the doctor who would recommend it, and, at least in most cases, only a downside for the mother and baby. (I acknowledge that there are some cases in which this type of intervention can be life-saving.) Although often downplayed as "routine" by medical providers, a C-section is *major surgery* and requires a much longer recovery time for the new mother. I had friends who discussed with me that they were still in pain over a month after the procedure as compared to others who had delivered vaginally and were back on their feet in a matter of days.

There has also been a rise in the U.S. in the number of women who chose to labor at home or to have a doula with them at the hospital to act as an advocate for their rights. When I first heard about this, I thought it was crazy! Having a midwife or doula with you for comfort or support is one thing, but why would an expectant mother need a third party present to ensure that her wishes were respected during her own labor? But the more I read and the more I heard from other moms, the more reasonable it seemed. There seems to have been a breakdown in communication with the medical establishment, and, from what I understood, the expectant mother needed to come into the hospital with almost a combative attitude if she was to have any say in her labor plan. One friend of mine who was set on having a completely drug-free delivery was actually mocked by the hospital staff who asked her, "Where are we—in a barn?" I also heard a personal story from a woman who was treated as an unwanted pest and almost brought to tears by a doctor's rude attitude simply because she wanted to interview him about his birth philosophy. For all these reasons, by the time we arrived in Spain, both Erick and I were very wary of any type of intervention and were a little on the defense ourselves.

Nonetheless, after much discussion and contemplation, Erick and I decided on Tuesday that I would go in for a scheduled induction on Thursday, August 5th. There were no signs that I was about to go into labor, but if I was going to be induced in a matter of a few days anyway because of health concerns, it made sense to go forward with the doctor I had come to know and respect, instead of a complete stranger. Our daughter was full-term and we could tell from the ultrasounds that she was a healthy weight. At that point, more time in utero would just have allowed her to gain more weight and increase the odds that there would be complications with the delivery. We had a choice between the 4th and the 5th. Since our daughter's middle name was to be Elizabeth, like her great-great-grandmother, we chose August 5th—Elizabeth's birthday in 1886. Until his death at almost 90, my grandfather (Elizabeth's son) always lovingly referred to her by her full name, *Clara Elizabeth*.

As an aside, the name Clara had been chosen just weeks before my due date. We originally planned to name our daughter Corinne. We even had a baby shower where that name was printed on the invitations. Once we realized, however, that friends and family were already misspelling and mispronouncing Corinne, we decided to go back to the drawing board. We set about finding a traditional and internationally recognized name that was easy to spell and pronounce in at least English and Spanish. Erick and I quickly realized that we each had different cultural associations to certain names. For instance, I liked Olivia, but Erick insisted that was Popeye's wife.

That is apparently her name in translated cartoons. In English, Popeye is married to Olive Oyl, not Olivia. (I also learned that the meaning of the name Popeye is likewise completely lost in translation.) We had such a hard time with this that we wondered how we would ever name another child if given the opportunity! Thankfully, the name Clara fit the bill and we both really liked it. Some of the grandparents had to warm up to it, though, since they all thought it was too old-fashioned. But, if we had started taking votes, I fear we would still be choosing a name. After Clara was born, we were amused by how many people from different backgrounds claimed that we had given her a Latin, French, Croatian or Catalan name! Our choice of Clara as an "international" name was apparently a success.

Now that we had a name and had scheduled the induction, and I could stop worrying about whether I would go into labor during rush hour and what that would be like in the back seat of a cab, I set about making final plans. I obsessed that we did not have just the "right" items from the hospital's list of things we should bring, but managed to pack our bags anyway. We also needed to finalize sleeping arrangements for Clara in our apartment. The rental office had offered a small portable crib so we went down the block to request it. I explained to the young woman in the office that I was all set to deliver the next day and, in response, she exclaimed in horror in her thick Scottish accent, "Oh my God!" I had spoken with this girl in person about ten times before. Had she really not seen this coming? She seemed in genuine shock that I was intent on going through with this whole baby thing.

Then, after we secured the crib, I went out for one more pre-labor walk along the beach. I watched the sunset over the city and said a prayer. I reflected on our time so far and how our lives were about to change forever. I couldn't wait to meet Clara.

B-Day

"Where there is love there is life." — Mahatma Gandhi

The delivery day had finally arrived. We got up early and there was a strange sense of calm, excitement and anticipation. We kept telling each that today was *the day*. That day was so strange for us. We were about to become parents for the first time and we did not know what to expect, to think or even to feel. Up until that day, we had been preparing for Kasey to start feeling contractions or for her water to break; we would have then called the doctor and gone to the hospital, but nothing so dramatic was happening. The day looked and felt like any other and Kasey was feeling as normal as ever. People were going to work on a typical Thursday morning. I could not believe that we were on our way to the hospital to actually have a baby, and all my thoughts were on Kasey and what she was about to go through in the labor process. The thought that Kasey alone was going to feel all the pain and do all of the work was making a knot in my stomach.

Kasey had been distracting herself with worries about packing the bag and reviewing the list of things that we were supposed to bring to the hospital. She repeatedly laid out Clara's clothes and everything else on the bed to make sure that nothing was forgotten. She was full of joy and trepidation, anticipating the next day when we would hold Clara in our arms for the first time.

I did not know how Kasey would react during labor. She was unusually calm and seemed a little checked out in my opinion. This was clearly out of the ordinary, but I figured it was her way of preparing for something unknown and scary. I kept praying for her and asking God for wisdom to do my part.

I knew that I needed to be there for Kasey and inspire in her calm and confidence. I knew that at some point, I may need to make decisions or speak for her. But no matter what happened, I knew that my role on this day would be miniscule compared to hers. I felt almost irrelevant. I was afraid for Kasey and wished that I could be the one delivering. I kept trying to put all those thoughts aside. I would concentrate on making sure that no matter how excited or worried I got that day, I would suppress my emotions for the time being and look only calm and reassuring for Kasey's sake.

We walked to the main avenue from our apartment as though we were just running behind for a doctor's appointment (we were about 30 minutes late). We grabbed a taxi and with no traffic arrived at the hospital in about 20 minutes. We walked into the administrative offices where hospital personnel pulled up our information. We were asked to sign only three pieces of paper in total (amazing!) to check in. One was a privacy notice, one was a bill for the hospital services and the last one gave the hospital staff permission to perform emergency procedures on Kasey or Clara should it become necessary. They ran our credit card for half the amount of the total bill. The other half of the bill would be paid when we checked out. We were surprised and amused when we saw an actual bellhop arrive (with pillbox hat and all) to take our suitcase to our room. We took with us only what we would need for the actual delivery, including a small baby blanket that would be Clara's first. The entire process took about 20 minutes and just like that we were all checked-in just like at a hotel. Another bellhop then took us down to the elevator and to the delivery floor that was located in the basement. This was the end of the familiar hotel experience.

We were shown into a small changing room that was reminiscent of a containment room from a virus outbreak movie. Another door opened and a nurse greeted us and showed us the locker where we could put our belongings and then gave us medical robes to change into. It was now very clear that we were in a medical facility about to have a very delicate and important procedure.

We were quickly introduced to our English speaking midwife who worked with the hospital. She contacted our doctor and got Kasey ready to be induced as planned. In the meantime, we saw the anesthesiologist walking into the room with a cart with all his equipment ready to place an epidural. We explained to them in English that although Kasey was being induced, she wanted to have as natural a birth as possible and intended to wait on the epidural until her labor had considerably progressed if she chose to use one at all. The midwife looked confused and insisted that Kasey get the epidural. I was thinking of all the stories we had heard back home where pregnant women ended up having procedures they did not want after arriving at the hospital. At this point, I became more protective and wanting to make sure there were no misunderstandings, I switched to Spanish and insisted that things would be done as we had agreed with our doctor. I noticed that the anesthesiologist looked uncomfortable, and feeling unwanted, he had started quietly moving his cart out of the room while I continued talking with the midwife. It was clear to me that she was upset that we were not letting her do her job, but I still made it clear that Kasey would not be getting the epidural or any other procedure until we decided otherwise. I also told her to call the doctor and she could then get the answers to any other questions she may have. She left the room and mumbled on the way out that this was not how things were done.

Our doctor arrived a few minutes later to say hello and we felt much better as soon as we saw her. She explained to the midwife our plans to do everything as naturally as possible and walked us again through the steps. First, a gel would be inserted that would help Kasey's contractions get started. Hopefully, the contractions would progress and Kasey would dilate enough to finally go into labor. As the doctor spoke with us, I saw the anesthesiologist taking his cart away again as he had been outside the room anticipating the doctor's instructions. At around 9:30 a.m. the doctor applied the gel. She told us she would be back soon to check on Kasey's progress.

Shortly after the doctor left, Kasey started having contractions. She had an external monitor attached to her belly, which was connected to a printer with a chart that went all the way up to one hundred where I could see the intensity of the contractions. The contractions were initially mild and about 10 minutes apart. The needle on the chart kept moving up to 30 or 40 with each contraction and Kasey seemed to be doing quite well.

After about two hours when the doctor returned, the contractions had not gotten much closer or stronger. The doctor then explained to us that since Kasey was not progressing, she could manually break her water or we could continue waiting. She explained that if she did nothing, Kasey could continue laboring like this for a very long time, but that nobody was in a hurry so it was up to us. She left the room to let us discuss it in private. We talked about it and decided to let the doctor go ahead and break Kasey's water. After the quick, but rather painful procedure, the doctor told us that she would be back in about an hour or when Kasey had dilated to at least 4 cm.

Soon after she left, Kasey started complaining about the pain of each contraction. They were much stronger now and I could see the needle on the machine quickly going up to the one hundred mark and way over! In a ridiculous attempt to be helpful, I started alerting Kasey when I saw the needle beginning to move. She quickly told me that she did not need me to tell her. She was *painfully* aware of when a contraction was coming. She was now crying and screaming with each contraction and they were coming one after another without any breaks in between. The midwife was clearly upset and I heard her exclaiming that Kasey did not need to go through all this pain during an induction and that this was completely unnecessary and she should have had the epidural from the very start. After Kasey had been having these very painful contractions for about 45 minutes, the midwife and another nurse that were never far away came to check how dilated Kasey was and both times she was still only at 3 cm. Kasey had screamed with every check and as they came to check her a third time I told them that I would not allow anymore checking and that I wanted our doctor to come down to the room.

The contractions kept happening back to back with no time in between for Kasey to breathe and prepare for the next one. I had been asking Kasey to tell me when she was ready for the epidural and now she wanted it. I ran out of the room and told the midwife that Kasey would be getting the epidural now. She told me that she did not want to get in trouble with the doctor and would call her and wait for her to come down. As I heard Kasey still crying in the room, I told the midwife that I would get the anesthesiologist myself if necessary as I would not allow my wife to be in excruciating pain for another minute after she wanted the epidural. As the midwife was about to go looking for him, I saw the anesthesiologist coming around the corner with his little cart, ready as always.

The doctor arrived only a few minutes later as they were preparing the epidural. It had been well over an hour since Kasey's water was broken and she had started screaming. I was desperate. She looked afraid and other than being able to hold her and keep her company, I felt completely impotent. I would have done anything to take her place.

The doctor checked Kasey and confirmed that she was about 4 cm dilated. She needed to get to 10 cm to deliver. The doctor was very comforting and encouraging. She helped Kasey calm down by holding her head and looking her straight in the eye while she told her that she understood her pain, that she had two children of her own and that this was what labor was like. She was very stern, professional and compassionate at the same time. I could see Kasey looking more composed and less afraid. This is when I realized that only a doctor she trusted, a woman and a mother could have comforted her at this moment. The doctor stayed with us while Kasey got the epidural and finally relaxed. The worst part was over. It was now early afternoon. The effects of the epidural were miraculous. I could see the needle on the chart go to one hundred every few minutes while Kasey was all relaxed and smiling. As the doctor assured me that Kasey would be okay for a long while before delivering I decided to go call Kasey's parents as I had promised.

Cell phones did not work in the basement so I had to change back into my clothes to go outside. I called Kasey's Mom first. Local time in S.C. was around 3:00 a.m., and she was half asleep and so anxious that she could not understand a word I said. I told her that Kasey was fine, but she kept repeating, "baby girl, baby girl" as I tried to tell her that Kasey had just received the epidural. She finally understood and thanked me for calling. She asked me to stay with Kasey and not worry about calling back until I had time.

Immediately after, I called Kasey's Dad who after hearing about Kasey asked me how I was holding on. Knowing his sense of humor, I told him that Kasey had me in a head lock for a while, but that I would be okay. I don't think I had ever made him laugh so hard. It was already past noon our time and after talking with Kasey's parents, I stopped to get a sandwich at the clinic's cafeteria (I would need my energy for the afternoon) and then hurried back to the delivery room.

Kasey was completely relaxed and resting while continuing to have contractions. I could not believe my eyes watching the needle on the chart going over the one hundred mark while Kasey was there pleasantly talking with me.

At about 3:30 p.m., the midwife came in to check Kasey's progress. She was now 10 cm dilated, but the epidural had begun to wear off. Kasey requested that she be given another dose, but the midwife advised against it out of concern that Kasey would not be able to feel enough to push. The doctor had also warned us about that possibility. Kasey was moved to the delivery room as the contractions were getting more and more painful. Kasey was crying again and I insisted that she receive another dose of the epidural. Just before the doctor arrived, the anesthesiologist administered another dose and Kasey began to relax. By about 4:00 p.m., it was time to push. The doctor had me stand behind Kasey and push her shoulders up with every contraction. I am not sure if I was helping Kasey at all or if the doctor just wanted to keep me busy after I said that I would not be filming the birth (although I had my camera with me, we decided to commit these private moments to just memory).

At around 4:15 p.m., as Kasey continued her final pushes, the doctor told me to come around to watch our baby come out. I declined saying that Kasey preferred I stay by her side (I could see plenty from where I was standing). She kept sounding very encouraging while telling Kasey that she was doing a great job. "Just one more," the doctor kept saying. By then, the midwife was on top of Kasey helping by pushing on her belly, but I could see that the baby was no closer to coming out than 30 minutes before no matter how hard everybody pushed. We had talked about not wanting an episiotomy unless the baby was at risk or Kasey was about to tear badly. The doctor and the midwife started to look concerned. The external monitor was showing the baby beginning to stress. The doctor reached for the scissors and gave me a stern look. As I nodded to her in agreement, the doctor proceeded to cut Kasey. Clara's head came out and she started firmly pulling her by the neck.

What a shocking sight that was for me! I was not ready for that and every protective instinct in me kicked in. For a second it did not matter how patient, wonderful and caring this woman had been. My only thought was that this stranger was cutting Kasey and pulling our baby by the neck like a chicken! I could see the doctors muscles tense up as she did it. I had to protect our baby I thought! I managed to restrain myself, although I felt enough adrenaline to tackle an entire football team. Yet, I was just standing there holding my camera in one hand. It felt so wrong. I should at least be doing something useful. I should be helping somehow. I knew that I should only watch and do nothing for now and I knew that I had to trust this doctor. This moment lasted only a few seconds, but it felt like an eternity. In her forcefulness, I could also see that the doctor was being very careful, and her face looked focused and confident. I did trust her, but I could not believe what was happening. I was still keeping my emotions in check, but I could clearly feel them bottled up inside of me, ready to burst out as soon as I let my guard down for a second. Then I saw this little human being coming out. That tiny person was my daughter being pulled out of my wife! Why was her skin purple? I could see the blood pouring out from Kasey's cut and the doctor removing the placenta. I understood and related to the stories of men passing out in the delivery room. I did not know how much more I could take.

I followed the nurse's every move as she took our tiny baby from the doctor's hands to the cleaning table. I could see the doctor applying the stitches to Kasey who looked relaxed as though she felt nothing. I hovered over the nurse telling her to be careful as she cleaned Clara. Clara clearly did not like what was going on and started to cry in protest. Her little cry immediately broke my heart. I wanted to hold her and comfort her, but I would have to wait another interminable minute. She stopped crying as soon as she was wrapped in her blanket. She looked healthy and was turning to a normal color now.

Now that everybody looked okay, I was finally able to take the first picture of our newborn. Clara was placed on Kasey's chest. Her eyes were now wide open looking at us while we introduced ourselves. She seemed curious and was paying attention to us while crossing her tiny hands. After the whirlwind of emotions I had been feeling that day, I was now just marveling at the site of my heroic wife and my baby girl. And, we were taking our first family pictures.

Participating in Clara's birth was the most intense, amazing and humbling experience I have ever had in my entire life. To see God's miracle of life and Kasey's courage in that moment is a memory that to this day gives me a knot in my throat and makes my eyes tear up in complete awe and admiration for her and mothers all over the world.

When Clara was born, *Bethel's* pastor was very eager to share the news with the congregation and even asked me for a picture of her to post on their website. He also added a note to their bulletin board welcoming little Clara into the world. At the same time, friends from our church in Fort Lauderdale sent us pictures of the flowers they had placed on the altar in celebration of Clara's birth. Kasey's Mom's Baptist church in South Carolina also made the announcement during their service. Like any other parents, we felt that our daughter's birth was a very important event. Including a close friend in Argentina, my parents in Venezuela and my brother and his wife living in Australia, Clara's birth was celebrated on four continents. Knowing that so many people in such faraway places were praying for her and celebrating her arrival only made it that much more special for us.

A Day of Firsts

"A grand adventure is about to begin." — *Winnie the Pooh*

After those first precious moments with Clara in the delivery room and after I breastfed her for the first time, I was wheeled back to our hospital room to begin my recovery. Clara arrived to join us after just a few minutes in the nursery. She had gotten all cleaned up and was a sight when we saw her! The nurses had dressed her in her tiny flowered onesie and had her lying on her side in a clear, portable bassinet cart. She was tucked in snuggly under a fitted hospital sheet and had a teeny light-green cap. Her multicolored, polka-dotted baby blanket was rolled up behind her as a back support. As I would later hear someone on the street comment, she looked as delicious as a *caramelito* (a little candy). Erick and I spent those first few hours marveling at Clara and checking her out from head to toe. We quickly decided she was perfect! I spoke with my parents and brother and shared in the joy of the day with them over the phone. Erick promised pictures just as soon as we got out of the hospital.

We were also taking stock of our room (where the bellhops had brought our luggage earlier in the day). There was of course a bed for me, but also one for Erick that the nurses made up for him each night. The hospital was situated on a hill so we had a window that looked out across the city to the Mediterranean in the distance. We had a private bathroom and the dinner that night was delicious (and healthy). I was actually given a menu with three options to choose from. My epidural wore off in a matter of a few hours and I felt pretty good. For the rest of Thursday and most of Friday, I stayed in bed, relaxed and worked on learning to breastfeed Clara. I was surprised when late Thursday night, about six or seven hours after Clara was born, my doctor called just to check on me and see how we were doing. Then, on Saturday morning before we left the hospital (and even though she was on vacation), she stopped by our room again to check on us one more time before she left town. She even gave us her cell number in case we needed to speak with her. I remain so impressed and grateful for her care and concern and the way in which she went above and beyond to help us have such a wonderful experience.

Later, when we went back for my six week checkup, I was happy to get a clean bill of health. While we were there, we could not resist asking my doctor to help us measure Clara as well. Thanks to the coin-operated baby scales at pharmacies all over town, we already knew she had a healthy weight gain, but we wanted to know her length. We laid Clara out beside a measuring tape and discovered that she had grown significantly. The doctor immediately commented, "Looks like she is going to be tall—like her mother." Erick, who is only slightly shorter than me, looked absolutely offended and without hesitation asked, "What do you mean, like her mother?" At first, before she realized he was joking, the doctor tried to hedge her comment, by saying that I was, "you know, really tall—for a woman." Erick started laughing. We would later hear those exact words many times and smile at the memory.

In addition to my doctor's visits, there were almost comical visits by the on-call hospital pediatrician. He would come in at various times during the day and, although I did not exactly understand what he was saying, stand at the foot of my bed, take out a chart from a stack his assistant was carrying, and give us Clara's "stats." Name, measurements, general health, and then off he would go to the next room. After a couple of these "updates," Erick and I had to laugh, but we were certainly happy that all reports were good!

It was also interesting for us to see that the "rules" of newborn care are not absolute. I guess this is not surprising since official guidelines seem to change a lot over time. For example, during my parents' generation, the recommendations in the U.S. were clear that a newborn was to be placed on her stomach to sleep. For my generation, this is a cardinal sin! It is almost considered child endangerment not to have a newborn sleep on her back. I was curious to see if the same was true in Spain, so I was amused that when Clara first arrived in our room, she had been placed on her side. As soon as we received her, we also placed little cotton gloves on her hands to keep her from scratching her face—as was customary in the U.S. The nurses were horrified and immediately insisted that we remove them. They were against hospital policy. Confused, we asked why. They explained that it was dangerous for the babies to ingest the fuzz from the gloves. Since that seemed reasonable, we agreed to forgo them.

My favorite memories of those first two days in the hospital, though, are of watching Erick and Clara as they began to bond as father and daughter. Before Clara was born, I had mentioned to Erick that he would enjoy dancing with his daughter one day. He was quick to tell me that it would be years before they would be able to do that. It was much to my delight, then, when on that first night, I caught Erick gently swaying with Clara to the quiet music we had playing on our iPod. It looked to me like was he was already dancing with his little girl and it was clear from his face that he was in love. He also recalls with great tenderness that first night when in between feedings, Clara used his finger as her first pacifier. He was head over heels and there was no going back.

Erick was also busying himself with visits to the nursery. Although Clara was staying with us in our hospital room (we chose not to let her sleep in the nursery) the nurses would come for her periodically to do checkups and so forth. Erick was intent on learning as much as he could from these professionals. After all, every time Clara came back from a nursery visit, she seemed calm and relaxed as though she had just been to a spa appointment. Whenever they took Clara, Erick would tag along and watch. Apparently he also tried on several occasions to coax his way into the actual nursery, but to no avail. He was restricted to the viewing area. Erick was also concerned that Clara's nose seemed too congested. Having had asthma as a child, he could not stand the thought that she was having trouble breathing. He kept insisting that the nurses come and clean out her tiny little nose and took careful notes each time. He was already so concerned for this precious little person who we would soon be taking home.

Two days later, it was time for me to check out of the hospital. I was feeling well enough to walk out by myself and was grateful for that. After we left our room, we realized that we would need to wait for a couple of hours to have one last blood test on Clara before she would be released to go home. We went down to the hospital diner with Clara and ordered some sandwiches for lunch. It was here that we received the first of several interesting "congratulations" gifts. The counter attendant at the diner clearly felt he needed to give us something to commemorate the occasion. He apologized for not having something more and gave us a handful of chocolates to celebrate! In the next few weeks, we would receive baby feeding spoons from the friendly lady who ran the store where we had purchased Clara's stroller, an adorable stuffed bunny from a friend at church and even a free onion from the man at the local vegetable stand! *Clara Catalana*, as the locals named her, received a warm and loving welcome to the world and to Barcelona!

That Saturday morning was a time of great reflection for me. Once Clara had the all-clear, we walked outside for the first time since she was born. It was a beautiful, warm, sunny day. We had planned to take a cab from the hospital back to our apartment. Every other time we had visited the hospital, it had been a weekday and the sidewalks and roadways were bustling with people coming and going from appointments. But since this was a weekend in August, there was no one around; just us standing on the curb with our tiny baby all wrapped up in her polka-dotted blanket. It was quiet and there was no distraction. After a few minutes, we asked the one passerby we saw to take our photo (with the compact underwater digital camera that Erick used for the entire trip). I love that photo that captured such a moment in our lives. We were newly minted parents just getting started on the real adventure of a lifetime! Erick went and asked the desk clerk whether they thought we should call a cab and they assured us that one would surely come in due time. We waited for another 20 or so minutes and a single cab finally arrived to drop off a visitor. We climbed inside to make our way back "home."

Our time in the hospital stood in stark contrast to other scenes I had participated in previously. Having grown up in a small community where most people had lots of family and friends nearby, when a new baby was born, many people (often dozens) would visit the hospital almost immediately after the delivery. On Friday, Erick tells me that our hospital was likewise filled with folks visiting the other new parents on the floor, most of whom who had gone home by Saturday. In the past, I too had felt that it was customary to visit a newborn baby before the family left the hospital. In Barcelona, of course, there were no visitors for us. For me, this was a preferable experience. I found that those first few days were filled with new experiences and that many of them were intensely private. I felt more comfortable having that time to recover physically and for Erick and I to bond with our new baby. We also found that we did not have as many health concerns for Clara because although we traveled a great deal in the first few months of her life, almost no one else handled her. So despite our having her out and about, she was not exposed to as many different people. I am not suggesting that everyone should (or would enjoy) being away during this time, but for me, it was a benefit that I had not fully appreciated before Clara was born. We decided that if we were blessed with another child, we would certainly do it the same way again.

All the Comforts of Home

"Home is where the heart is." — Pliny the Elder

When I would visit the hospital for my pre-labor checkups, my doctor would advise that should I go into labor naturally, it would be best for me to wait as long as possible before coming into the hospital so that I could labor "in the comfort of my home." Erick and I took one look around the hospital and laughed. There was no comparing the "comforts" of our tiny rental apartment with the comforts of this world-class clinic! We would just come in straight away, we thought.

But the physical comforts of our home away from home aside, of the many benefits we enjoyed on this trip, the one that cannot be overstated is the special family time that we would have missed almost entirely had we remained in the U.S. We had certainly considered this aspect when we decided to go abroad, but since we had never had a newborn, we could not have appreciated just how wonderful having Erick at home would be for our new family. First, if we had stayed in Florida, in all likelihood, I would have worked right up until the day I gave birth. For me, this meant that instead of spending my days walking around Barcelona, taking afternoon naps, getting into better shape and studying Spanish at my leisure, I would have been commuting almost an hour each way to and from my office in downtown Miami in heavy traffic and then sitting all day at a desk where I no doubt would have just gotten even fatter (did I mention I gained 50 pounds anyway). Although I will never know, I have to wonder if my health or Clara's delivery would have suffered as a result.

If all went smoothly, though, and I avoided a C-section, I would have probably delivered at the local hospital and would have gone home to our apartment when Clara was about three days old. Erick would probably have taken off that Thursday and Friday to be with us in the hospital and would more likely than not have been required to go back to his office on Monday. He would not have been allowed to work remotely for any real length of time had we remained in Florida. Erick could have, of course, perhaps taken a few more vacation days that next week, but the societal expectation is certainly that the new mother (if she works) will stay home for about three months on unpaid maternity leave (if she is lucky) and the new father will return to work as soon as mom and baby are out of the hospital and situated at home. My parents would have come to visit for a few days and then returned to S.C. My Mom is a teacher and would have just been starting her school year so she would not have missed work. Most of my local Florida friends either have jobs or have small children themselves. Erick would have left for work around 7:00 a.m. and not returned until at least 6:00 p.m. at an office that, with traffic, was also almost an hour away from our home. Consequently, I would have been at home basically on my own. I am sure this is the unenviable situation for many working families in the U.S. Our situation in Barcelona, however, was completely different.

There is a prevalent cultural view that just because you are a woman, you must instinctively know how to care for a baby. I can tell you I did not, and I am going to go out on a limb here and suggest that *lots* of women, on the day they return from the hospital with their newborn, are equally clueless. Perhaps anticipating this revelation, when we went to visit some friends in the hospital about a year before Clara was born, the new mother said, "I can't believe they are going to let us take this baby home." Erick replied in jest, "They are not going to let you, they are going to insist!" I think perhaps many new parents feel that way though. I mean, you have to take a test to be allowed to drive a car and you are required to get a license just to be able to fish, so how can it be that we are entrusted with a fragile new life without any oversight whatsoever? But the fact is, we are, and I for one am eternally grateful to have had a partner at home with me for the first two months of Clara's life to help navigate the ups and downs of this new, life-changing experience.

Since we were in Spain, although Erick was working, he was *there* day and night. In between conference calls and emails, he changed diapers and did feedings. I want to note here that I am intentionally not saying that Erick "helped" me because that would imply both that Clara was my primary responsibility and not ours together, and it would undermine Erick's role in her life. He did not, and does not, "help" with Clara, but is completely involved as her father. But more important than the physical support I had with Erick at home which is, in and of itself, pretty important to a tired new parent, we were able to figure things out together. Erick had considerably more experience than me with a baby simply because he was old enough to remember what it was like when his younger brother was born and his insights in general were invaluable. As a new mother, I of course, was also recovering from the physical trauma of labor and delivery in addition to trying to learn to breastfeed which can be exhausting and frustrating especially at first. To this day, I believe that Clara was a calmer, happier baby in large part because she had two loving parents there to care for her instead of just one overtired, and inexperienced me.

Having Erick there during those first months was also wonderful for me on a personal level. I am the kind of person who gets cabin fever easily and who craves conversation and interaction. Had I been confined to my home alone for several weeks or months, I think I would have been in serious danger of experiencing some level of postpartum depression. Obviously, that would not have been good for anyone involved. So having

Erick, my husband and best friend, there with me during this time was just incredible. And, it was not just having Erick there for the hard parts of being a new parent that was so wonderful, but having him there for the high points! He did not miss any new "coo" or have to wait to hear things second hand from me. Instead, we were able to share all those precious first moments together as a new family. And, as I mentioned, I could not have fully understood the impact this one facet of our decision would have on this experience, but looking back, it was indeed the greatest gift of all and would be reason enough to do it again.

Succeeding and Breastfeeding

"True humility does not know that it is humble. If it did, it would be proud from the contemplation of so fine a virtue."
— Martin Luther

One of the major lessons I learned on this adventure was that I needed to relax and not give myself such a hard time about "succeeding." Many expats who have chosen to relocate to another country will probably agree that humility is key, especially when you don't speak the language and when you are (way) out of your comfort zone. For me, in addition to being a temporary expat learning to function in a different culture, and in a foreign language, I was also learning how to be "mommy" to my beautiful little girl. In the interest of full disclosure, I had about *zero* prior experience with children when Clara was born. I had not had baby siblings and had never even babysat before I was due to be in charge of this precious newborn. Aside from what I had read or seen on television (and the information provided by the clinic in a very cute ten page illustrated instructional guide), I was basically clueless. As many new parents may relate, it frankly seemed almost insane that I was allowed to leave the hospital with such a delicate child. I was, however, extremely fortunate to have a dedicated partner who was and is completely invested in our parenting journey.

Erick and I were in agreement that I would breastfeed Clara for as long as it was possible to do so, but for at least the first few months before I returned to work. We both felt it was the healthiest option for our newborn. Before our trip, I read books and articles about breastfeeding and tried to learn as much as possible. I even went to the breastfeeding class at our local hospital in the U.S. It was clear to me from all my studies that this was a natural process and that it would, therefore, come naturally to me. Sometime during this process, I also apparently came to believe that this was an integral part of motherhood and that "failure" was not an option. Unfortunately, I was in for a rude awakening. Clara and I started out pretty well in the hospital and it seemed that she was latching on and that we were both getting the hang of things. My doctor stopped by the day after I delivered and gave us some more tips. When we left the hospital, I thought all was well. We had no Plan "B" and because of the things I had read, I did not want to give Clara any bottles or a pacifier for fear that she would then refuse the breast.

Around day four, after we were settled back in our apartment, the trouble really began. That afternoon, Clara began crying inconsolably, which she had not done since she was born. Since I was exclusively feeding from the breast, I had not been able to measure how much milk she was taking in. I knew that I was trying to feed her every few hours, but now she was struggling to latch on. I became increasingly frustrated and upset. At first, we thought maybe she had gas (which seems to be the one-size-fits-all answer anyone at a loss will give you when a baby is crying). But eventually, we decided the situation was out of control, and since she was so little, we decided to go to the emergency room. Once we declared ourselves in an "emergency" situation, Erick sprang into action and rushed us out the door. We hurried down the stairs and jumped into a cab to go just two blocks to the local public hospital. I was still a little (okay—a lot) emotional and not quite recovered from the delivery. I was crying myself when we arrived at the emergency room door. In that moment, I was sure that I was not fit to be a parent. Here was the proof. Erick spoke with someone at the front desk and we were immediately brought inside to a patient viewing room. Although we were not officially residents of Spain (just being there as tourists), and because a child's access to health care is considered a human right, they accepted our daughter into the public hospital without any paperwork. Just minutes later, a considerate young female doctor arrived to see

Clara. The nurses also came by to console me. The doctor checked out Clara and determined that she was in perfect health—she was just hungry!

The doctor gave Clara a bottle and "prescribed" several ounces of milk every three hours. When she heard us discussing whether or not to use a "pacifier" she laughed. It was apparently the first time she had heard the English word and was insistent that yes—it would *pacify*! The doctor also told that us that she regularly saw newborn babies come into the emergency room dehydrated, which she attributed to an over-emphasis on the importance of breastfeeding. Apparently, like me, despite the potentially dangerous consequences to a baby's health, many new mothers are hesitant to supplement with a bottle. Although I was still concerned that because of the bottle, Clara would not now be willing to breastfeed at all, I was beginning to realize that my attitude about the whole thing was very unhealthy, unnecessarily stressful and more than a little nutty. I just wish I could have seen that *before* our trip to the ER. If I were going to dispense advice to new moms, it would be that it is great to have a plan, but remember to be flexible! After this incident, I bought a breast pump so that I could measure how much Clara was taking in from me. I had to supplement with formula, because despite lots of pumping and many more attempts to feed Clara directly from the breast, I never produced anywhere near enough milk. I continued to pump for the next two months mostly just to give Clara whatever benefit she might be able to get from even a small amount of breast milk. In hindsight, I am not sure that I would have tried to breastfeed exclusively anyway, though, simply because of the exhaustion factor. We also got Clara a pacifier and she did not have any trouble switching back and forth from the breast to the bottle.

I would also like to add a little note here on the ER we visited. I know for some people, the words "public hospital" conjure up unpleasant third world images of overcrowded and understaffed facilities. To be clear, this was not the case at all. We had actually visited this hospital once before when I was still pregnant. Although I was sold on the private clinic on the day we meet our doctor, Erick insisted on shopping around so we went to check it out. We vehemently tried to find someone at the public hospital who could give us a quote for the delivery cost, but everyone we spoke with insisted it was free. We were certain this could not be the case for us because we were not Spanish citizens, but we never quite got to the bottom of it. The only downside that we could see as far as labor and delivery was that during my recovery, I may have had to share a room with another mother. By coincidence, we also spoke with a young first-time mom who worked with our apartment rental company who had nothing but good things to say about her recent experience giving birth in the public hospital. When we were there "shopping," one physician even offered to examine me right away because she seemed to think that I may not have ever been seen by a doctor (despite my obviously advanced pregnancy). We assured her that I was okay and ultimately decided that we would stick with our first choice. After our ER trip with Clara, we were also surprised to find that, within a few days, we received correspondence mailed from the hospital that had a detailed breakdown of the "treatment" provided to Clara and the recommendations from the doctor. We joked that it basically said, "Infant will be fine—not so sure about mother!"

Call Me Ishmael

"What's in a name? That which we call a rose
By any other name would smell as sweet."
— William Shakespeare, Romeo and Juliet

Once Clara was born, we needed to get her a passport so that she could fly back to the U.S. In the U.S., hospitals provide the birth certificate, but in Spain, the midwife provides a form that one must use to get the baby registered with the civil authorities. We needed this registration for the American Consulate to give us a Consular Report of Birth Abroad, which we could then use to acquire Clara's American passport.

I was not sure what to expect from the Spanish bureaucracy. I looked for directions to the Civil Registry closest to our neighborhood and it was relatively nearby. Once I arrived there, I only waited about three minutes before someone helped me. I asked what I needed to do to get my newborn registered and they gave me a one page form to fill out with Clara's information. It took me one look to realize that I was going to need help with even the most basic questions. It required me to fill out the parents' names and places of birth, national ID numbers and address. This was very simple, straightforward information for anyone else maybe, but not for me. I had been given a number and was supposed to have the form ready when called. Five minutes later, my number was called and my form was empty.

I started by telling the lady that called my number that I needed some help filling out the form. She looked puzzled, clearly thinking I must be illiterate or very dumb. She politely asked me what help I needed. I told her I needed help with my name. You can imagine the look she gave me.

Let me explain why. In Spain and in Venezuela (as in all of Spain's former colonies), everyone has a name, a middle name, their father's surname and their mother' surname, in that order. Therefore, my "last" name in the U.S. is actually my Mother's surname, and not my Father's. Also, in Spain, women do not change their last names when they marry; they always keep their maiden names and pass it on to their kids. Therefore, Clara, being born in Spain, would have automatically gotten my first surname (not my "last name") and Kasey's last name. Since Kasey had dropped her maiden name altogether and taken my last name when we were married, in Spain, using our American IDs, Clara might have gotten my last name twice (once from me and once from Kasey). If this form was not filled out correctly, Clara could also have gotten my Father's surname and my Mother's maiden name or even my last name as a middle name and Kasey's middle name as a last name. None of this made any sense in Spain or in the U.S., but we were caught in the middle of two different naming conventions and I needed to make sure that our child got it right.

In trying not to look so crazy, I started sharing things with the clerk that I had learned over time such as that in Portugal and Brazil children always get their mother's last name. In the Netherlands, it is tradition for children to get all four of their grandparents' first names and their father's last name, and in Greece, the children get their father's last name, but it is spelled and pronounced differently depending upon whether the child is a girl or a boy. I do not think that any of this trivia made me look any better. After all, it was completely reasonable to expect me to know my *own* name and be able to write it on a form. The lady that had been so patiently listening to me was still just looking at me and the empty form now sitting on her desk.

She finally figured that she would just ask me to tell her what I wanted my child's full name to be. Yes! I knew that for sure.

Clara Elizabeth Prato, I said with excitement. Although, from her point of view, my daughter was getting her grandmother's maiden name and neither of her parents' surnames (which I am sure is a travesty no matter where you are from), she did not judge. She simply asked me to write it down and proceeded to add a note to the registry saying that the baby was getting only one surname according to personal legal right ART 219 RRC.

After ten minutes, we had everybody's names sorted out, but had completed only the first line. The rest of the form remained empty. She asked what else I needed help with. Nationality/place of birth and address I said. I was sure that she would lose her patience with me then and think that I was just trying to be difficult. I proceeded with more explanation. You see, my place of birth is Venezuela and although my child was born in Barcelona, we really live in Florida and my wife and I are Americans, but we need our daughter to be registered in Spain in order to get her American passport.

She told me that she would need to talk to somebody about this. I was sure at this point that she would call security. To my relief, she just confirmed with the lady at the desk next to her which countries to use and two more lines in my form were filled out. We were making progress!

Then, the form asked for my family book, so I asked what that was. In Spain, they have something really neat. When two people get married, they become a family unit and they get something called the *Libro de Familia* (Family Book). This book looks like a really big passport and has information about the whole family, including the names of the parents of both the spouses. It also has pages for any children that may be born to the couple.

It turned out that to register Clara, I needed to register myself and Kasey first and start our Family Book. This required all of our information including our names, surnames, address, nationalities, both of our parents' names, our marriage certificate and the date and place of our marriage. This book needed to be obtained in another office. I asked for directions to the other office and headed there by myself, without wife or child, with just two passports, a note from the midwife and a lot of explaining to do.

I will simply sum it up by saying that after visiting two government offices that were within walking distance and waiting no more than five minutes in each before being helped, I was able to get everything I needed for all of us to be registered with the Spanish government, and was successful in obtaining the document that the American Consulate required for Clara's passport. And, despite the unique challenges that I/we presented, I was amazed by how cordial and understanding the public Spanish employees were. All was done properly and it took me just a couple of hours.

I was elated by how well and easy everything had gone and we figured that getting Clara's passport would be a breeze since we were just requesting an American passport for the child of two American citizens.

Becoming American

"A certificate of live birth is not the same thing by any stretch of the imagination as a birth certificate." — Donald Trump

Now that Erick had secured the necessary documentation from the Spanish government, we needed to set about making Clara "official" in the United States. But first, I enjoyed getting to explain to my parents how it was that they were now documented in the official records of Spain. They had not seen that coming for sure. When I explained the concept of the Family Book to Mom, she exclaimed with glee that she was now "just like a *conquistadora!*" I guess there were some unexpected benefits even for Mom. But nonetheless, we needed to have Clara recorded with the U.S. authorities as well as the Spanish.

We wanted to get started with this process early so that we would have Clara's passport in hand by the time we planned to return to Florida. There was no urgency for our local international traveling, though, since we would not be flying. So when Clara was about three weeks old, we gathered all the documentation and took a cab over to the U.S. Consulate. There is only one U.S. Embassy in Spain and it is located in the capital, Madrid. An Embassy generally houses a high-ranking diplomat that may serve as a spokesperson for a national government abroad. A Consulate, on the other hand, is a smaller establishment that houses a Consul, or lower-ranking diplomat, who is charged primarily with assisting expatriates with issues they may encounter abroad. For example, in Barcelona, with its common petty theft, many of the Consulate's "customers" appeared to be unwary tourists who had lost their passports and needed replacement documents to return home to the U.S. And then of course, there were people like us, who were temporarily or permanently living in Spain and who needed U.S. documentation of some kind.

The U.S. Consulate building is itself a striking presence and was a bit of a surprise to me. It is in a beautiful part of the city, high up on a hill and surrounded mostly by quiet, almost suburban streets. But despite its location and peaceful surroundings, the Consulate is completely encased by high concrete walls and looks more like a compound than an inviting public space. In order to go inside we had to pass through an outer and inner guard station and then go through a process that resembled airport security. They also took our cell phones and held them until we were ready to leave. I was not expecting quite this level of security in Barcelona, where there are hordes of tourists each year and no apparent threats. Having said that, however, everyone working at the Consulate was courteous and (mostly) helpful.

When we arrived, we first needed to get a passport photo for Clara. Fortunately, on site, they had a small photo booth for just this purpose. Inside the booth, the instructions said that the person should position their head so that it was reflected in the circle on the screen. As you might imagine, this was a bit tricky as Clara was sound asleep and, of course, otherwise rather uncooperative. After some maneuvering, Erick finally managed to get a clear photo of Clara's head with his hand holding her up, but her sleepy little eyes remained closed. We then took our documents and photos to a waiting room where we filled out a few additional forms. We gave all the necessary documentation, including both of our U.S. passports, to the counter clerk. She first told us that Clara's photo was unacceptable because her eyes were closed. We looked at her a little incredulously and explained that Clara was three weeks old. She said she would check with the Consul. After a brief wait, she returned and explained that the photo would be fine, but that we were missing our original marriage certificate. Of all the things we thought we might need for this, our original marriage certificate had certainly never crossed our minds.

We explained that we did not have it and would not be able to get it before we needed to travel back to the U.S. She then brought over the Consul to speak with us in person and despite our explanation of the situation, he *insisted* that we had to have our marriage certificate because it was on the list of required documentation. To us, this was just crazy because we were *both* U.S. citizens and under the rules, had we been unmarried, either of us could have registered Clara. Since this was the case, we suggested that perhaps I alone could register Clara now without the marriage certificate and then Erick and I would sort it out when we got back to Florida. The Consul refused, insisting that since we had already indicated on the form that we were married, we would have to produce an *original* marriage certificate. He suggested that we have someone in Florida send it to us. We explained that we did not have any family in Florida and that no one else even had a key to our apartment. And even if they had, I was not even sure where to tell someone to look for it and I recalled how difficult it had been with the delivery service before. After we made it clear to the Consul that there was no one who could retrieve this document and that it was simply not an option, he went so far as to suggest that one of us would need to fly to Florida and bring back the certificate before Clara could leave the country. Which of us should go I thought to myself sarcastically, the breastfeeding mother or the only person who was fluent in Spanish? He could not be serious, I thought.

At this point, Erick decided to call the Consul's bluff since it was clear that he had simply dug in his heels and was going to refuse to back down on this ridiculous issue. I was beginning to get upset, but I kept thinking there was no way this person was actually going to deny a passport to the newborn baby of two U.S. citizens. Erick asked the Consul if he would please write a letter stating that he had denied Clara a U.S. passport because she did not have the requisite documentation. As Erick understood it, under Spanish law, if a child born in Spain had no right to the passport of any other country, the child would be entitled to a Spanish passport. He thought that if the Consul would give us some proof that he would not issue her a U.S. passport, then we could get her Spanish passport immediately and work out any issues with her U.S. documents once we returned to Florida. Aside from the red flags we might raise at the immigration check points on our way back into the U.S. with different passports from that of our newborn, we were confident that we would have no problems getting Clara's U.S. passport once we were back in the U.S.

Clara was a U.S. citizen from the day of her birth regardless of where she was born. Unlike a foreign national who moves to the U.S. and later becomes a citizen through the naturalization process, Clara is a "natural born" U.S. citizen because she is the child of two U.S. citizens and she never held a different citizenship. In other words, as inspired by the great American author and fellow South Carolinian, Stephen Colbert, one could say that Clara simply needed to "re-become the American she never wasn't." Although to my knowledge, the U.S. courts have never addressed the issue head on, as far as I can tell, she should even be able to run for president of the U.S. one day should she so choose. I'm sure it would make for an interesting cable TV pundit debate though.

Of course, the Consul refused Erick's request for a written denial because it was obvious to everyone that he was being completely unreasonable and, as I suspected, he knew his position was indefensible. Instead, to save face, he said that he needed to "run it by" the D.C. office and that it would be a few days before we could get an answer. But he did agree to take all of our signed paperwork and hold it until he got the okay to process it. About three days later, we received the call that all was well and that we could pick up Clara's passport in a matter of weeks. Erick was bummed, though, because he had begun to hope that they would deny our request, which might have opened the door for Clara to get both passports almost immediately. Two weeks later, we returned to the Consulate and obtained Clara's Consular Report of Birth Abroad, which is the effective equivalent of a U.S. birth certificate, and her passport. Now, not only was Clara logged in the official records of Spain, but she was all set for her first international flight to the U.S.!

Kingdoms and Castles

Baby Steps

"Make voyages. Attempt them. There's nothing else."
— *Tennessee Williams*

After three weeks of breastfeeding/pumping for Kasey, both of us getting up every few hours during the night (our place was way too small to avoid everyone waking up every time Clara was hungry) and me working from 2:00 p.m. to 11:00 p.m. every day, we were exhausted with the routine and anxious to go on a trip! As eager as we were to travel, we wanted to take a short test trip first to see how much of a traveler little Clara was. At the car rental office, I remembered having seen a beautiful poster of a cold looking place in the Pyrenees called Andorra, and since we were in the middle of a hot summer, nothing sounded better than going to the mountains. After looking it up on the map, I learned that it was only three hours away by car. I knew nothing about Andorra, but quickly did a little research online to learn a few things about our next destination.

Andorra is a small independent country, famous for its ski resorts, spas and shopping streets. Only two and a half times the size of Washington D.C., it is located between Spain and France. It is part of the EU and part of the euro zone, and the local language is also Catalan. However, 70 percent of the population is foreign (mostly from Spain, France and Portugal) therefore all four languages are widely spoken. It looked to us like the perfect short trip.

I booked a hotel and a car rental online on Friday during my lunch hour, and after finishing my work day at 11:00 p.m., I stayed up late hand drawing a map with directions to our destination (since I still believed that no international GPS was available at the car rental closest to our apartment). The next day, after waking up every three hours for Clara's feedings, I was exhausted but still managed to leave our place by 10:00 a.m. It was a hot and sunny Saturday in August. I walked to the metro station and in 30 minutes was done picking up the car and on my way back to get Kasey and Clara. Even though I had reserved the least expensive car available (about $50 a day), to my surprise, I got a brand new car with A/C, power everything and a manual transmission (most Spaniards do not like automatic transmissions and they are hard to find at rental places). The best and most distinctive feature for us was the windshield. It went all the way back to the middle of the roof past the driver's head and could be covered like a moon roof. I had never seen one like it before, and it was the perfect car for sightseeing as we were headed for the mountains on a sunny and cloudless day. I was very excited with our little, but very cool car and thrilled with the way our day had started. After getting back to the apartment and sharing with Kasey the great news about the car, I carried our small suitcase and stroller to the car (now feeling like such a dad!). Kasey carried Clara and celebrated with me the amazing view we would have. We started securing Clara's seat/bed in the backseat for the first time and confirming that everything was hooked up properly so that she would be safe and comfortable. Just 45 minutes later, off we went, very excited to take Clara on her first international trip!

The trip was supposed to take three hours, but we stopped several times to take pictures of the beautiful scenery and to feed and change Clara. Kasey was riding in the back seat with her and Clara seemed to be enjoying the ride as much as we were. She was either sleeping or pleasantly resting while mommy looked over her. The drive through the mountains was phenomenal, and with very little traffic, I was really enjoying driving a manual transmission. Getting to the hotel was very easy (even with the great map I had drawn half asleep in the middle of the night). It was helpful that there was only one road in and out of Andorra that crosses the country from Spain to France.

We arrived at the hotel in the afternoon. In my reservation, I had neglected to mention that we had an infant, which distressed the very friendly manager. After admonishing me for my lapse in providing such important information, he quickly moved us to a bigger room and offered us a pack n' play for Clara to sleep in at no additional charge. After some breast pumping, feeding and another diaper change, we were ready to stroll around town. The hotel manager was very worried about Clara and pointed us to a restaurant across the street. Other restaurants in his opinion were too far for us to walk with a stroller. After warning us about the terrible drivers and the traffic, he urged us repeatedly to be careful pushing the baby stroller on Andorra's "dangerous" streets. We found this very humorous since there was only one two-lane road. Living in South Florida, with its notoriously aggressive drivers and overcrowded highways, which we took every day to work, to us, Andorra was extremely peaceful in comparison. After promising to be careful, we disregarded the advice from our very concerned hotel manager and started walking directly toward the downtown that was only a few blocks away. *Andorra la Vella*, the capital of the principality of Andorra, is the most picturesque city. It sits in a small valley, surrounded by beautiful mountains and is crossed in the middle by a river. Its downtown is full of trendy shops and plazas and its cool weather makes it a great place to walk and stroll around in the middle of the summer. We were pleased to see that Clara was also a hit among the Andorrans who couldn't help complementing her everywhere we went. We spent the day marveling at the scenery and taking pictures in town. The next day, we went to other nearby ski towns that even in the middle of the summer were full of tourists enjoying themselves. We decided that we needed to come back in the future, maybe in the winter, and enjoy one of these resorts. We had a lot of fun with the street signs around town, which always pointed to Spain in one direction and France in the other (just taunting me I was sure). Kasey kept joking about wanting to drive just far enough to cross the border into France both to appease me and to take Clara into her third country at just three weeks old, but unfortunately, we didn't have quite enough time.

On the way back from Andorra, Kasey wanted to drive. She had not driven in Europe yet and she was eager to get behind the wheel of our cool compact car. Kasey was thoroughly enjoying the drive through the Pyrenees; so much so, that since I was distracted with Clara in the back seat and not paying attention to my flawless map, once back on the Spanish side of the mountains, we missed our exit to the highway and stayed on the old two-lane windy road for an extra hour. Once we missed the exit, it was impossible to switch drivers on the narrow road and since Kasey did not have that much experience with a manual, by the time we found another exit to the highway, she was more than a little tense and white knuckled from gripping the stick shift. In hindsight, and despite her trepidation on the road, we agreed that the drive was so spectacular that we were quite happy to have taken the long detour.

Since we had taken a different route back, we drove all around the city before getting to our neighborhood. We were only about 15 minutes away from our place when we realized that it was almost time to feed Clara and we were out of milk. The idea that Clara would cry from hunger when we had no food in the car was horrific to us as brand new parents. I was thinking that we would be the worst parents ever, even if we were only unable to feed her for 10 minutes. We almost went into panic mode. We had gotten used to being able to feed Clara on time and she never cried for longer that it took us to get her bottle ready. I started questioning the whole trip, thinking that it had been a terrible idea. Thankfully, we made it home by around 10:30 p.m., just in time to feed Clara before she even fussed.

That night, I still needed to return the car. I had rented it until Sunday, and the subway that I needed to get back home closed at 11:00 p.m. I rushed to the car rental office that was only 10 minutes away by car, but I didn't know that it was closed on Sundays. I left the car across the street and dropped the keys in a box they had for such purpose. I took the subway home where Kasey was already back to her pumping routine and Clara was happy and rested. Our great weekend and first family trip had been saved from a last minute "disaster" in just the nick of time!

A Shrine to Laziness

"You must avoid sloth, that wicked siren." — Horace

When we first began strolling around Andorra, we saw an imposing structure in the middle of the city that we could not quite identify. Its glass paneled peaks were gleaming in the late afternoon sun and it looked like Superman's Fortress of Solitude or something else out of an otherworldly sci-fi thriller. It stood out in stark contrast from the rest of the architecture in the city. We started discussing what it could be. Maybe it was a new-age church with a giant steeple, or perhaps a hotel or maybe just a monument meant to imitate the surrounding mountains? After we got closer, our curiosity was killing us and we had to get inside. To my great amusement, it was an enormous spa!

When I was growing up, my Dad was obviously an influential person in my life. He has always been hard-working, entrepreneurial and eager to try new things. He almost always has a new project in mind and is not one to rest on his laurels. In fact, I think I probably got my sense of adventure and curiosity from him. And, although he has built some beautiful places in the Carolinas, I sometimes suspect that having always been in the construction industry, his idea of relaxing is building a new place to relax. I am also pretty sure that among the seven deadly sins, Dad would rank sloth right up at the top. I wondered then what my Dad would think of this hedonistic palace, which Erick and I immediately dubbed the "Shrine to Laziness"!

Once inside the *Caldea* (Google it—it is really something else), as it is called, we passed several shops and then entered the center of the building where we took an elevator to the top floor observation deck. We watched as the sun was sinking below the mountains and decided to stay and have dinner in the restaurant that overlooked one of the huge soaking pools below. As we took our seats and ordered our meal, we could see that just above the surface of the water, there were several white flying-saucer-like jacuzzi bowls filled with relaxed tourists. In addition to this central area, which even had a laser light show in the evenings, there were both indoor and outdoor areas where all manner of treatments could be enjoyed. I love the idea of a spa and this one was really over the top. Although we could not go in ourselves (because I was still recovering from labor and we had Clara and because it had not occurred to us to bring our swimsuits to the mountains), we declared it one of our top places for a second visit in the future.

The Land of Don Quixote and Wine

*"Do you see over yonder, friend Sancho, thirty or forty hulking
giants? I intend to do battle with them and slay them."*
— Miguel de Cervantes Saavedra, Don Quixote

Labor Day weekend was coming and with me taking one
additional day off from work, we would have a four-day
weekend for our next trip. After our successful trip to Andorra
with Clara, it was time to go back to France and Kasey was eager
to visit the wine valleys of Bordeaux. We would take a different
route this time. Instead of crossing into France along the
Mediterranean coast, we would head west from Barcelona
through the Spanish wine valleys toward the Basque region and
then head north and cross into France along the Atlantic coast.
We would then head back east through France and return to
Barcelona along the Mediterranean. I made reservations online
for two nights in a hotel just minutes outside Pamplona and for
two nights in the French city of Bordeaux.

As I researched our route, I learned fascinating facts about
the areas we were about to explore. Our drive would take us
out of Catalonia through Aragón, Navarra and the Basque
region. These regions of Spain are the vestiges of what had
been independent kingdoms in the not so distant past. These
places are so unique in their history and identity that they have
their own distinct ancestral languages that are still widely
spoken today. Although these ancient kingdoms have since
become part of what we now know as Spain and France, this
fact has only added Spanish and French to their linguistic,
historical and cultural diversity.

In just a four-hour drive, in addition to the Spanish and
Catalan languages, we would also encounter Aragonese,
Euskara and French. While the others are Romance languages,

Euskara has no connection to any other language in Europe. Also called Basque, it is classified as a language isolate. It is the last remaining descendant of the Pre-Indo-European languages of Western Europe and, to this day, its origins remain somewhat of a mystery to linguists and historians alike.

As usual with my busy schedule at work, on Friday I was still drawing maps with directions to the hotels until well past midnight. On Saturday morning, we were ready and eager to go. We left our place planning to be back by Wednesday, on time for me to start working at 2:00 p.m. The weather was perfect when I went to get the rental car. Kasey and Clara were ready when I got back to the apartment and we quickly left Barcelona taking the highway headed west.

Our route was full of historic sites with medieval towns, castles and remnants of Roman Empire era aqueducts and theaters, which were all perfectly blended into the awesome landscapes with beautiful valleys filled with sunflower plantations and grapevines alongside the road. Modern infrastructure was the norm along our route and I was particularly fascinated by the many modern wind turbines that could be seen along the Spanish highways in these regions.

Having recently read *Don Quixote* (considered to be the first modern European novel), I was very aware that these were the very lands where the comical knight had his misadventures tilting at windmills. We made many stops along the way to take pictures of the impressive landscapes and the modern descendants of the giants that inspired Miguel de Cervantes four hundred years before. However, these particular giants looked to me much more like the also impossible to vanquish three legged Martian machines of H.G. Wells than the traditional windmills of *Don Quixote*.

Right at dusk, we arrived at what was supposed to be a very good, but inexpensive, hotel on the outskirts of Pamplona. Since online pictures of hotels can sometimes be deceiving, we were never quite sure how reality would compare to our expectations. We were pleasantly surprised to see that our hotel was even bigger and more beautiful than the pictures led us to believe. It was built with all the charm of a mountain cabin, but with all the comforts one could possibly want. As we explored the hotel, we were even lucky enough to enjoy watching a wedding reception from one of the wooden terraces.

The next day, we rested in the morning and then asked the hotel staff about local attractions. They showed us pictures from a tourist book of the region with several interesting places. We decided to head toward a town only half an hour away called Olite. We were simply expecting a nice little town where we could stroll around and have lunch. But, once again, reality greatly exceeded our expectations.

The medieval town was beautiful and incredibly charming and as we approached the city center, we began to suspect that something special was going on. We soon realized that we had arrived right in the middle of their annual *Fiesta de la Vendimia* (Grape Harvest Festival). There were hundreds of people celebrating, live musicians, folkloric dancers, stands with typical food and wine dealers from all over the world. There were wines from dozens of local wineries for all the visitors to taste (for free) and delicious foods and *tapas* being sold at the main plaza. Since Kasey was still breastfeeding and would not be drinking wine, she loved that in the center of the plaza they also had stands with different rows of grapes for tasting. Each batch of grapes was labeled with the particular variety of wine that it produced. She enjoyed sampling the precursors to the region's best wines: Cabernet Sauvignon, Merlot, Garnacha,

Tempranillos, Mazuelos, Gracianos as well as the Viura, Chardonnay and Garnacha Blanca.

Our surprise was complete when we saw from the plaza the very imposing *Palacio Real* (Royal Palace). Olite, even though a small town now, had been the seat of the Royal Court of the Kingdom of Navarra in the Middle Ages. Its palace was home to monarchs and princes and with its impressive Gothic architecture, it was declared a national monument in 1925 and is now open for visitors. The Royal Palace was built in the 13th and 14th centuries and was turned into a luxurious palace in the 15th century by the King of Navarra, Charles III "the Noble." The palace was built next to an even older castle built two centuries earlier, which had been converted into an upscale hotel.

We decided to participate in the ongoing celebrations first and visit the palace later in the day. Clara was charming the locals as usual while enjoying the music in the sunny but cool weather. After drinking and eating to our satisfaction, we proceeded to tour the palace that occupied no less than one third of the old medieval town. The inside managed to exceed everything I could have imagined from its outward splendor. It was right out of a fairytale and it took us over two hours to see it all. From the highest tower, we enjoyed a magnificent 360 degree view of the surrounding area. We were clearly in wine country. Grapevines and wineries could be seen all around while dozens of wind turbines dotted the hills in the distance. Olite turned out to be a fantastic recommendation and a great example of why it is always a good idea to ask the locals where to go. The next day, we planned to visit the city made famous by Ernest Hemingway in *The Sun Also Rises* and walk the very streets where the Running of the Bulls takes place every year during the *Fiesta de San Fermín* (we did not quite make it in time for that festival in July, which is probably all for the best).

I neglected to research in advance the city of Pamplona and did not have a plan for where to go or what to visit; therefore, we drove around first to get a feel for the city. We were now in the Basque region and the architecture, although still Spanish, was different from that of Barcelona and the other cities we had seen closer to the Mediterranean. The city seemed somewhat more compact and the otherwise common balconies and terraces were hardly noticeable here. Walkable areas were still abundant as in any other city we had seen in Europe. We quickly found convenient parking and started our stroll around the city, visiting the parks, plazas and historic sites. People would also stop us here to complement Clara in the warm and friendly manner that we had seen everywhere else in Spain.

I should mention here that the work schedule and meal times in Spain are quite different from the U.S. (especially in the hot summer months). Since we arrived in Spain, we had noticed that at noon restaurants are closed. Before 2:00 p.m. (when Spaniards have their lunch), one can only find open the occasional *tapas* bar or coffee shop. Having become such fans of the *tapas*, this served us quite well though. We were beginning to get used to the streets and plazas being pretty much deserted from 4:00 p.m. until around 6:00 p.m. when people avoid being outside in the heat, and even most stores remain closed. Since we continued having lunch around noon though, adapting to the late dinner time was much harder for us. Many restaurants only start to serve dinner around 9:00 p.m. and most do not fill up until much later. Main streets and plazas, where many restaurants are located, also fill up with people for these late night outings.

After refreshing ourselves back at the hotel during the afternoon, we went downtown for dinner. At around 9:00 p.m., we arrived in one of the main plazas, which was full of families with their kids enjoying their summer break. As we had come to expect, the restaurants were only beginning to set the tables for dinner. As we picked a restaurant and ordered our food, Kasey was excitedly talking about everything we had seen during the day when she complained that I was ignoring her. I was completely mesmerized by a table directly behind her.

She quickly forgave me when she turned around to see what had captured my attention. Two couples had just arrived (past 10:00 p.m.) with eight kids ranging from one to about eight years old. When I saw the waiter arrive with the drinks, I pointed out that there were no crayons, no toys and no plastic cups! Every child got the same breakable glass that you would only serve to an adult, the sodas were still in the cans and the kids were about to serve themselves. I told Kasey that since I joked about wanting to have eight kids, I needed to pay attention to this show. I was expecting a major train wreck and could pay attention to nothing else. We speculated about what could possibly have possessed these two couples to say to each other, "Hey, let's go out to dinner with all of our eight little kids. What a great idea! That sounds like fun. See you at the plaza at 10:00!" And, that they decided to do so unarmed with any toys or other distractions.

While seeing families out with kids this late at night was completely normal in Spain, we had never seen this feat performed in such numbers. While all four adults were never seated and eating at the same time for more than a few minutes (one was always chasing one kid that had run away into the plaza), to my surprise, they all had a remarkably pleasant and civilized time. This event did not seem to be a one-off crazy night never to be repeated. They seemed to have done this before and were quite competent at it. No glass was broken, only one toddler cried for a few minutes and only one drink was spilled. The most amazing part of this sight was to see how the parents were actually enjoying themselves as well as the kids well past midnight. I had found new heroes.

The next day, we were ready and eager to continue our trip. Our route would take us very close to the city of San Sebastián (in Spanish) or Donostia (in Euskara), the capital of the Basque region. I confess my ignorance here by saying that all I knew then of the Basque country was from immigrants I had met as a child while still living in Venezuela. I knew that many Basque did not consider themselves Spanish at all, and I had also seen news reports of the occasional actions of the small but violent separatist group E.T.A. that wanted independence from Spain at any cost (a large number of regional Basque representatives on the French side have similarly lobbied to create a Basque department, to no avail so far).

I had seen on the Spanish map that San Sebastián was crossed in the middle by a river that ended in the Bay of Biscay in the Atlantic Ocean. I figured that any European city with such a geographic location had to be worthwhile visiting. My curiosity about the city and its mysterious language made it imperative that we stop at least for lunch before entering France.

Unbeknownst to us at the time, San Sebastián is one of Spain's most famous tourist destinations. Despite the city's relatively small size, major events such as the San Sebastián International Film Festival have given it an international dimension as well. San Sebastián, along with Wrocław, Poland, will be one of the European Capitals of Culture in 2016. The architecture, while still clearly European, looked neither Spanish nor French to me. The city was a very different place and with the public signs in Euskara, it felt like we had jumped over to a place as far away as Russia. Only the fact that Spanish was still widely spoken gave away that we were still on the Spanish peninsula. With its own unique charm and colorful buildings, I suggested to Kasey that being only 45 minutes away from France this city may have been a better choice for our maternity leave. But while she was happy to visit San Sebastián, Kasey's heart was still in Barcelona.

Being in such a beautiful city, we lingered much longer that we had first intended and strolled around the delta and the boulevards where I kept finding irresistible picture opportunities everywhere I looked. After spending a leisurely afternoon with our one month old daughter and eating some of the local food, we reluctantly continued on our way toward France.

Sleeping Beauty

*"Let us step into the night
and pursue that flighty temptress, adventure."*
— *J.K. Rowling, Harry Potter and the Half-Blood Prince*

As we crossed the French border, the highway started gaining altitude and the valleys of Spain gave way to a dense forest that reminded Kasey of the Carolinas. It was still daylight when we arrived in the city of Bordeaux, yet, the city looked gray and run-down. We were relieved to find our hotel quickly and pleased that it looked as good in person as it did in the online pictures. However, the street in front of it was deserted and the neighborhood looked dark and unfriendly. After checking in and relaxing for a little while, I was eager to go back to the town for a second look. Kasey was tired and decided to relax at the hotel with Clara while I went to practice the very little French I had managed to learn since my misfortunes during our first trip to France.

Bordeaux was a completely different city at night. It really lives up to its nickname of *"La Belle Endormie"* (The Sleeping Beauty). The buildings were lit up from the bottom and what had looked to us like a gray, uninviting place just a few hours earlier now looked like the most fabulous destination. The city is divided by a large river and after much driving I finally found a parking spot on the main boulevard by the river bank. I left the car ready to take great night pictures and enjoy some fine French cuisine. Being by myself, without having to push a stroller or be mindful of diaper changes and bottles, I figured that I would be able to cover a lot of ground. Although they had given me a map at the hotel, I didn't think I would need it and simply made a mental note of the car's location.

I started walking without a clear plan looking for good places to photograph. It was taking me forever to find the proper settings on my camera for the poor light conditions when I realized that my camera's battery had died. I continued walking the streets, still trying to recover from the deep disappointment of not being able to take more pictures of this "sleeping beauty." Suddenly, it started to rain, and in a matter of minutes, it was pouring and I found myself running for cover. The streets were now deserted and most businesses and restaurants had closed for the night. After about an hour, it finally stopped raining, but it was now very late, I was wet, I had no pictures and I was hungry. I kept looking for an open restaurant and the only place I could find was a fast food burger place. Having run out of options, I had one of the combos with a Coke, which I was able to order without problems since I now knew the numbers in French. Out of shame at having eaten a cheeseburger combo during my night out alone in France, I kept this part of my story a secret from Kasey for a few days.

After finishing my shameful combo meal, I decided to call it a night and go back to the hotel, but I quickly realized that I could not find my way back to the car. I looked for the map I had gotten from the hotel clerk, but I must have lost it while running in the rain. I figured I would practice my French and ask someone to point me toward the river where I had left the car. The only issue being that after all the rain, and with everything closed, there was no one around to ask. I walked back to the burger place and it had now closed as well. I finally found some people and asked them for directions to the "river," but they did not seem to know what I was talking about. I started to doubt that I was saying "river" correctly, but I was pretty sure. I kept walking and looking for someone else when it started pouring again. I was now completely soaked and very annoyed. When it finally stopped raining, I saw several guys entering a little door by the side of a building into what I thought had to be a night club. I followed them in to ask for directions and soon realized that it was a gay bar.

So much for my plans of taking great night pictures of the city of Bordeaux while enjoying good wine and sophisticated cuisine. Instead, there I was, drenched at two o'clock in the morning, in a gay bar, lost and asking for a river in French that did not seem to exist. At least these guys were quite friendly with me and after much effort, one of the guys finally exclaimed something in French that sounded to me like "the canal" (a completely different thing that no one could have inferred from my asking for a river I guess). After being pointed in the direction of "the canal," I finally found the car—only four blocks away.

I arrived at the hotel in the early morning hours to find Clara and Kasey pleasantly dreaming and completely unaware of my misadventures. I would wait for a better time to tell Kasey about my foolish night. The next morning, Kasey gloated (just a little) that she, on the other hand, stayed dry and had eaten a delicious meal of meats and French cheeses in the hotel lounge while enjoying the company of some very friendly Canadians who had also fallen in love with our daughter.

Cheers, *Salud, À Votre Santé*!

"Beer is made by men, wine by God." — Martin Luther

When we woke up the next day, I was (relatively) rested and ready to go out and explore the famed Bordeaux wine region. After Erick told me a little about his night, and we had a good laugh, we headed down to the hotel lobby to investigate our options for the day. I found a *very* large book on the hotel coffee table with listings for nearby wineries that we might be able to tour, but the choices were utterly overwhelming! It seemed there were hundreds of places one could visit and I had no idea where to begin. Since we had had such good luck before with Olite, we decided to once again ask a local for guidance. The desk clerk suggested that we go to the nearby town of Saint Emilion. Although I've no real basis for comparison in the region, in hindsight, I am confident that this was a great decision.

After a short drive through some of the most beautiful landscapes we would see during our time in Europe, we arrived at the outskirts of the town. There were vineyards as far as the eye could see and I felt truly transported to another time and place. I later learned that Saint Emilion is a UNESCO World Heritage site with a history that dates back to pre-Roman times. Vineyards were planted there as early as the 2d century and stunning Romanesque cathedrals make up the skyline. The town was named after the monk Emilion, a traveling confessor, who settled there in the 8th century and the monks were apparently the first to begin commercial wine production in the area. Erick was like a kid in a candy store that day with his camera (now fully charged).

Saint Emilion is filled with quaint restaurants, layered terraces that overlook the vineyards below, and, of course, enticing shops where you can walk in and sample the local wines. When we arrived, we parked our car in a small lot just outside the town and walked into the first open building we saw. We were greeted by an English speaking young man who was eager to share his knowledge of the region and his love of the art of winemaking. We found it curious though when he informed us that he "did not drink alcohol, only wine." While many might classify wine as "alcohol," here the distinction suddenly seemed very important. We lingered in the store listening to his explanations of the winemaking processes and tasting various local creations. We decided on a favorite and bought a few bottles to take home.

When I mentioned to my Dad that we were going on this trip and that we would be visiting the Bordeaux wine region, he requested—only somewhat in jest—that I learn how they grow the grapes so that he might give it a shot in South Carolina. Dad has a small vegetable garden and recently constructed a wine cellar under his house and since, as I mentioned, he likes to try new things, I promised I would look into it. When I mentioned to the young wine broker that my father might be trying his hand at winemaking, he encouraged me to send him a bottle as soon as it was in process. I don't think I acquired enough expertise on this trip to see much success in bottling my own vintage, or enough to help Dad out with his endeavor, but it is always nice to know that we have a potential buyer!

After packing our bottles back in the car as well as the stroller, which we quickly realized could not handle the cobblestone streets, we returned to explore the rest of the town. Clara relaxed in the chest carrier while we walked around the narrow streets and spent the afternoon soaking up the ambiance of this age-old place. It was arguably my favorite day of the entire trip. The slow pace of the town allowed us to really appreciate the beauty of our surroundings and I found that it was an excellent place for some quiet personal reflection. Near the end of the day, we circled the town in our car and continued to enjoy the scenery as the sun set in the distance.

We then returned to Bordeaux, refreshed and ready to re-experience the city. Despite Erick's previous misadventures, he had continued to rave about how beautiful the city was at night and insisted that I go out with him to see for myself. We drove into the city center and he was absolutely right. The lit building facades and the cathedral in the main plaza looked incredible. We found a small restaurant and sat outside to enjoy a delicious meal at the end of our picture-perfect day.

After having had a relaxing and wonderful trip in the wine regions of Spain and France, we headed back eastward across southern France. This route would take us right past Toulouse, a city Erick had seriously considered as a home base for our time in Europe. He was still lamenting not having had time to stop for a visit, when about two and a half hours outside Barcelona, we saw a huge fortified city off the highway. This was obviously a place that we needed to visit and we made a mental note of the approximate location to look it up later.

The Best Laid Plans

"It is good to have an end to journey toward; but it is the journey that matters, in the end." — Ernest Hemingway

After having satiated my urge to visit France for a little while, we remained as busy as possible exploring and enjoying the many sites of Barcelona. Even after two months, we still felt that we were barely scratching the surface of what the city had to offer. We visited the aquarium near our apartment (the biggest in Europe), the Magic Fountain of Montjuic, the *Parc de la Ciutadella*, the Royal Plaza and the *Plaza de España* and walked and dined in many of Barcelona's distinct neighborhoods. I couldn't believe that Kasey even eagerly hiked through the imposing hills of Park Güell just a few short weeks before her due date! We enjoyed several local festivals (I'll let Kasey elaborate on those) and kept trying the seemingly endless choices of delicious foods and pastries. Even though we still had a list of places that we wanted to visit in Barcelona, the travel bug had bitten us and we had just one more opportunity for a longer trip before we had to return to Florida.

This would be our last and final trip before going back to the U.S. and I finally allowed myself to take two days off. Since Clara had done so well on our two previous trips, we would take advantage of her good traveling disposition and go farther this time. Our ultimate destination would be Geneva, Switzerland and, if possible, the town where my last name originated in Italy, Prato. Geneva was about eight hours away by car. Because of Clara, we would continue to obey our self-imposed limit of no more than three hours in the car at a time, which meant that we would make several stops along the way there and back. The plan was to leave early on Saturday morning and return on Wednesday by 2:00 p.m. local time (8:00 a.m. in Florida), just in time for me to check back in for work.

Choosing the route was easy. We had looked up the medieval walled city that we had seen from the highway on our trip back from Bordeaux, and Kasey found out online that it was Carcassonne, a fortified city founded by the Visigoths in the 5th century, which had been thoroughly restored in 1853. It had also been added to the UNESCO list of World Heritage sites in 1997. According to its website, it was a hub for the rich and famous, especially during lunch time on Saturdays. It was therefore clear that we would be having lunch in Carcassonne on Saturday. From there, we would take the fastest route toward Switzerland, drive around Lake Geneva, cross into Italy through the Alps and come back to Spain along the French Riviera. I took my honorary role of travel planner very seriously and created spreadsheets with the details and activities. Kasey, as my number one client, was very pleased and excited when I showed her the trip itinerary and quickly exclaimed her motto since we got off the plane in Europe: "This is the way to spend maternity leave!"

Although this would be our last chance to make it to the town of Prato in Italy, which had no particular interest to us other than being our family name, going there would have added six hours to our trip and an extra day and night we didn't have. The family pictures next to the Prato signs would have to wait for another time in the future. We would still have the opportunity to stop briefly in Genoa, though, where my great grandparents were from. I was so obsessed with working remotely that it never crossed my mind to take an extra day off work and we didn't want Kasey to miss another day of class, but, in hindsight, we absolutely should have done it.

Our stops would be as follows without driving more than three hours in between: Carcassonne and Mornas in France, Geneva in Switzerland, the *Castello di Pavone* and Genoa in Italy, and finally Monaco and Cannes before returning to Barcelona.

As had become my routine before going on a road trip, I was busy drawing maps at midnight after working until 11:00 p.m. Kasey had the night shift with Clara while I tried to get some good sleep before the drive the next day. On Saturday, I left for the car rental place early. It was cloudy and rainy (not a good start for a road trip). I was hoping to get the car with the panoramic windshield and we were lucky! This was enough to make me forget the lousy weather and how tired I was. By 10:00 a.m., we were on our way to France (which always made me very happy). The plan was to leave Carcassonne by around 5:00 p.m. in order to look for the hotel while we still had daylight. Hopefully, Clara would then let us have a good night sleep before heading toward Geneva the next day.

By the time we arrived in Carcassonne, it wasn't raining anymore and the weather got progressively better throughout the day. The medieval town was completely spectacular with 3 km (1.86 miles) of walls from late antiquity. Massive defenses encircle the castle, the surrounding buildings, its streets and its fine Gothic cathedral. The town history was fascinating. The earliest known occupation of the site where the town now stands dates from the 6th century B.C. Absorbed by the Roman Empire in the 1st century B.C., it came under Visigoth rule in the 5th century. It was taken by the Arabs in 724 and reconquered in 759. The city went through many sieges, wars and revolts until the mid-1800s when restoration efforts finally began.

We spent the day learning about its history, walking around and taking some of the best pictures of our whole trip. If you like photography, history, castles, fortresses, cobblestone streets or anything medieval, do not miss out on visiting Carcassonne if you ever have the opportunity.

Clara enjoyed the day as much as we did and we ended up lingering much longer than planned—again. As though we weren't late enough, when I saw the sunset as we were finally leaving, I had to stop to take one last set of pictures of the magnificent walled city. Kasey humored me and waited patiently while I drove around the city looking for a good hill where I could set up the camera. After taking the perfect picture of Carcassonne under the sunset, we were finally on our way to Mornas around 7:00 p.m.

Damsels and My Distress

"The gentle reader will never, never know what a consummate ass he can become until he goes abroad. I speak now, of course, in the supposition that the gentle reader has not been abroad, and therefore is not already a consummate ass. If the case be otherwise, I beg his pardon and extend to him the cordial hand of fellowship and call him brother. I shall always delight to meet an ass after my own heart when I have finished my travels."
— Mark Twain, The Innocents Abroad

Mornas was a completely random town that I picked online (without knowing anything about it) for the sole reason that it was midway between Carcassonne and Geneva. I found an inexpensive hotel next to a medieval fortress that seemed to have some character, however, it was off the main road and I was a little concerned that I would struggle finding it at night in the middle of nowhere. Since it was off the beaten path, it wasn't likely that I would find anyone who spoke English or Spanish if I needed any help.

Once again, my maps hand drawn in the middle of the previous night seemed to lack some detail and I did have trouble finding the hotel. However, we finally arrived around 9:30 p.m. The person at the front desk didn't look very happy to see me there and was trying to explain something to me in French. Eventually, the hotel owner came out and told me in English that they only accepted guests until 6:00 p.m. and that this was not "that kind of hotel" (as in a normal hotel, I thought). She was still giving me a hard time when Kasey walked in with Clara. As soon as the lady saw Clara, she forgot why she was mad at me and started talking about her grandkids and how cute Clara was. Then she started giving me a hard time again for not mentioning in the reservation that I had a baby. Thankfully, Clara came to my rescue again and stole all of her attention by making "goo goo" sounds. From that point on, the lady was as nice as she could be. She moved us to a bigger room on the upper floor away from the other guests in case Clara cried during the night.

The hotel had a lot of charm and character and was next to a medieval fortress. It was owned by a couple that lived there and they maintained it themselves (therefore the limited hours and different rules). The owner asked us about our trip and began telling us about her daughters that lived far away in interesting places like New York while she was still stuck in Mornas running the hotel. She repeatedly offered to take Clara for a few days until we got back from our road trip, and I think she really would have. She then showed us up the stairs to our room. Now that we were friends, and I was enjoying the conversation, I noticed that Kasey had gone very quiet, and was staring mistrustfully at the armored statue on the landing of the narrow stairway. Kasey is not fond of arms, or old or dark places. I was, however, quite amused with our very likely haunted hotel.

Kasey, Clara and I were hungry and while Kasey started feeding Clara I found out that the hotel restaurant closed at 10:00 p.m. The car tank was almost empty and I decided that it would be best for me to fill it up before the morning. I went out looking for fuel and nourishment. Everything was deserted, with no stores or even road lights for miles around. Finally, I found a gas station but it was closed. I tried a couple more that were self-service, but my American credit cards wouldn't work. I was dangerously close to running out of gas while still looking and decided to wait until the next day when the manned gas stations opened. The only open place for food that I found was a Middle Eastern joint. I went in and ordered two chicken kebabs with Mediterranean sauce. With my broken French, I got two hamburgers wrapped in flat bread with mayonnaise and French fries stuck in them. I was embarrassed just thinking of how I would explain the results of this foray to Kasey.

When I got back to the hotel, it was closed. *Closed!* All the lights were off and a metal fence that I had not seen before had been locked, completely blocking the access to the courtyard that led to the reception area. All I could see through the fence in the dark were two big dogs guarding the courtyard. There was no bell to ring or intercom button; only a keypad to introduce a code that I didn't have.

I was thinking of what to do. What if I found no way to get in? Even if I guessed the code to enter, how would I get past the guard dogs? Would I have to sleep in the car? Should I be eating while I thought about all this? What if Kasey worried herself sick waiting for me? I didn't know what to do and it was only getting later, I was getting hungrier and the food was getting colder.

Before leaving the hotel, I had briefly looked out of our room window to admire the fortress on the hill, and I remembered that it had a view of the side street. I walked around the building trying to recognize the window. Maybe if I hit it with rocks Kasey would hear me and look outside. There were several windows and they all looked the same. If I threw rocks at the wrong one maybe someone would call the cops and I would be taken to jail before anybody understood what I was saying. Who knows what kind of horrible food stuffed with fries and mayonnaise they would give me in jail? Would they even feed me in a French jail? Did I mention I was hungry? I decided to take my chances with the rocks. I never thought that I would complain about this, but Mornas had the cleanest streets I had ever seen in my entire life! Not a pebble to be found for blocks;

no sticks, nothing to throw at a window. How could the society that engendered the French Revolution have come to this? After half an hour of looking, I was about to throw the bread with mayonnaise, fries and all at the window when I noticed a tree with some kind of little fruits that I thought would make ideal projectiles. I looked at my watch and it was almost midnight. After foraging from the tree, I had a decent arsenal of projectiles ready. At the turn of the hour, I would begin my attack on this fortress. I hoped that the damsels in the tower would notice my distress!

It was pitch dark when I started throwing the little hollow fruits and they barely made a noise. I was beginning to think that I had the wrong window when I saw the face of a woman sticking out of my target. She looked scared and annoyed. I was sure that *gendarmes* would arrive next with sirens wailing.

It was Kasey! I told her that *They* locked me out. She asked me what I wanted her to do. She said that everything was dark and nobody was around, but that she would try to open the front door. I figured that if I had to, I could sleep in the car, since at least now Kasey knew where I was and I could finally eat. I walked back to the front of the hotel and waited for Kasey to come out. The dogs saw me this time and came out barking. A man then started yelling from inside in what sounded to me like Spanish, so I yelled back in Spanish. I then realized that it was French. I had nothing—so I yelled back in English. He finally came closer to the door and did not look happy at all. He started interrogating me in French. I had no idea what he was saying, but I could well imagine. Who the hell are you? Why are you here in the middle of the night? I will set the dogs loose on you and call the police!

While I was embroiled in my confrontation with the night sentinel and his dogs, Kasey must have been mustering the courage to walk through the dark by the armored knight standing on the stairway. As things got worse with my adversary, all of a sudden, I saw Kasey's head sticking out of the reception door into the courtyard. She had Clara in her arms and when the man saw them, he understood we were together. He finally let me in after telling me another thing or two while pointing at his wrist watch.

In the morning, I was eager to leave Mornas before I was admonished by the owner for waking people up in the middle of the night, but breakfast was included and after our disappointing dinner, I wasn't about to miss out on that. We spent some time talking with the nice owner who did not give me a hard time about the night incident. She kept offering to keep Clara for a few days as she explained to me that this was a family run hotel and that the man that let me in the night before was her husband. The dogs were just their harmless pets. After having a delightful breakfast and saying our goodbyes, we were on our way to Geneva before noon.

Power and Luxury

"Riches don't make a man rich, they only make him busier."
— Christopher Columbus

So far, we had been able to cross international borders without ever stopping or showing our passports to anyone. Since Switzerland is not a formal member of the European Union, though, I wasn't sure how entering the country would work. They also use the Swiss franc instead of the euro. For these two reasons, I decided not to get a hotel in Geneva just in case we had some kind of delay crossing the border. To be safe, I made a reservation just outside the border crossing on the French side (where I felt so comfortable and knew that nothing could go wrong).

Despite my planning, I missed a turn when I was looking for the hotel and, before we knew it, we were already in the very real border crossing with Switzerland. The French police were on their side and asked me to stop. I said *"bonjour"* and showed them the address of the hotel to ask for directions. They told me while pointing to the Swiss police and looking at them with unfriendly eyes (ten feet in front of us), "Tell the Swiss that I said you need to cross the border and then turn around and reenter France to get to your hotel." Although Kasey has chastised me in the past for unnecessarily "antagonizing" authority figures, this was one of those times when I could not resist. I drove the ten feet separating us from the Swiss guards and told them that "the French" had instructed me to tell them to let me turn around and follow their directions to our hotel. The animosity between these guys was obvious. The Swiss guard looked annoyed at the French and told me in perfect English that I didn't need to do that and that I could continue driving into Switzerland and take the next right to get to my hotel. Since we were on Swiss soil, I followed his instructions and in three minutes we had exited Switzerland another way and were back in French territory. After finding the hotel, we checked in and rested for about an hour before going back to Geneva to explore the downtown and have dinner.

I had never been to Geneva and for me the city was a symbol of cosmopolitan elegance, world-class luxury and power. Numerous and varied international organizations are headquartered in Geneva and I was very curious about the city. In reality, Geneva was indeed beautiful and organized and many of the main streets were lined with top brand stores. I joked with Erick that I didn't want to miss the chance to open my very own Swiss bank account (with the approximately 5 Swiss francs I had on hand). While in Geneva, we visited many of the famous landmarks like the *Jet d'Eau* (one of the world's largest water fountains) and the *L'horloge fleurie* (at one time, the largest flower clock in the world). And the night we arrived, we settled in at a beautiful torch-lit restaurant by the water in the city center. We decided to splurge a little on dinner as we reasoned that we did not know when (or if) we'd ever be back in Geneva. The terrace atmosphere was romantic and the ambiance suited all of my preconceived ideas about the city. Erick was also enjoying his opportunity to eavesdrop on the nearby tables where he could hear several different languages being spoken and was busy admiring our waiter who was taking orders in English, French, Italian and German.

Just as I was getting comfortable and really beginning to relish this luxurious dining experience, I smelled a strong stench coming from the stroller where Clara was now wide awake and looking at me. Clara and I politely excused ourselves to go to the ladies' room, but when I saw the narrow staircase that led to the bathrooms downstairs, I returned the stroller to the table and carried Clara down without it. Once inside the bathroom, I noted that there was no changing table and nowhere except the sink countertop to change Clara. I was alone in the restroom, so I decided to go ahead and try to change her quickly. Once I opened her diaper, however, it became apparent that this would not be so discreet. In my short time as a mother, this may have been the stinkiest, messiest diaper I had yet encountered. My luxurious euphoria from a few minutes before was quickly being shattered by my new reality. Thankfully, I managed to change the diaper before anyone joined me in the bathroom. I cleaned the countertop and then threw the diaper in what I thought was a trash can. I then washed my hands (not easily as I was still holding Clara) and reached for a towel. It was then that I realized that I had thrown the world's stinkiest diaper into the linen bin with the nice white hand towels. I quickly pulled out the bin, retrieved the diaper and moved it to its rightful place all while juggling Clara. Finally, Clara and I were refreshed and ready for dinner, but I was quickly learning that sophistication and decorum do not always flow seamlessly once you have a newborn!

While in Barcelona, a new friend that we had met at church, who had grown up in Switzerland, had recommended that after visiting the city of Geneva we should go to the *Château de Chillon* by Lake Geneva. We were still marveling that we were in Geneva and talking about how fortunate we were that the weather had been so great when we arrived at the *Château*. I had very low expectations from the word *Château* (I though it meant some kind of cabin). I'm glad that Kasey insisted on going. The *Château* turned out to be an awesome medieval castle with a breathtaking view of the lake. I got excited as soon as I saw it. I eagerly parked the car on the side of the road and immediately started walking toward the main entrance looking at the lighting from the sun and wondering what setting to use on my camera. Once inside, we started walking around and doing the tourist thing, reading the history of the place from the brochure and taking pictures.

The lord's quarters made this place quite memorable for me. They had the history of the owners over the centuries and explanations on how they had lived, and even many of the original household items. I think that the romantic idea that the royalty of old had wonderful lives is completely debunked once you see the "bathrooms" they had to use. I couldn't help but compare their lives of "luxury" to ours and see how much better off we were.

I particularly liked the maps (they looked about as good as my midnight drawings) with the routes and itineraries that the lords of the castle at different times would have taken in order to visit their domains. It took them weeks to cover the distances that we could drive in just hours with our baby, and they did it in uncomfortable carriages. We had air conditioning, a radio and a panoramic windshield. They needed hundreds of men and horses just to carry the possessions they "needed" for the trip. We just needed a suitcase and a stroller, and everything fit in the trunk of our little rented car that we didn't have to worry about. Of course, being that rich and with so much stuff they also needed an army to come along for protection whereas we felt pretty safe driving around with just a few euros in cash, some credit cards and a cell phone.

By any standards, these medieval lords were incredibly wealthy and powerful. Still, it was undeniable to us that we had luxuries and comforts they could not even imagine and could never have afforded (for example, A/C and disposable diapers). We had the incredible *power* to do things they could only dream of, such as the ability to travel comfortably at amazing speeds. We also have devices that could have only been described as magical like refrigerators, TVs, cell phones, cameras and computers. We have wonderful bathrooms, vaccines, epidurals and the Internet! And if all that wasn't enough to make you feel rich and powerful, you can add to that the fact that we enjoy all these things in relative peace and safety and with an unprecedented freedom that the old royalty never knew.

For many days after that visit and every time I remember it, I just feel so amazingly blessed and fortunate not only for where we live, but mostly for *when* we get to live. I think that wealth and power are usually, and unfortunately, associated to *privilege,* as in the things one can have and do that others cannot. I think real power, though, is the ability to accomplish something good and real wealth is not lacking the things that one *really* needs.

As if our visit to the *Château de Chillon* wasn't enough to make us feel privileged, the very same day we continued our trip toward another castle. This time we had a reservation to spend the night. After only three more hours of majestic scenic driving around the breathtaking scenery of Lake Geneva and then through the equally magnificent Alps and Aosta Valleys in Italy, we arrived at the *Castello di Pavone* around 8:00 p.m. on Monday. Among its illustrious lineage, this fortified castle had even belonged to the Pope and served as his residence at one point. It is considered one of the most beautiful castles in Italy and it has been restored and turned into a hotel (just for our enjoyment, I'm sure). Once again, I was elated. I did not expect much from my $150 a night reservation, even though it was well over what we normally pay for hotels. But, for a castle, I was willing to pay it for one night. For an additional $60, they included a three course dinner and a private tour of the castle. They treated us like royalty and the meal was a delicious feast with a bottle of wine and dessert included. Kasey and I enjoyed a romantic dinner while our baby daughter quietly looked around the intimate candle-lit dining room. We got a huge room with a modern bathroom and a jet shower. Kasey and I spent at least an hour each enjoying this much appreciated luxury away from the "comfort of our home."

Kasey and I kept appreciating the fact that we were not only more fortunate than the royalty of the past, but that we could literally enjoy the same privileges in a real castle. More importantly for us, we could do it for just a night and leave without having to own it, maintain it or, more importantly, defend it.

After dinner, I was eager to go take more pictures and tour the castle on my own. It was already midnight and although she was enjoying the experience, Kasey let me walk around by myself in what she described as the "dark, creepy" castle. She preferred to stay in the room with the doors well locked. When I told her about my night adventure walking around without a soul in the eerie dark hallways and chambers of the castle, she was quite happy to have missed out. She was even happier that she intentionally waited until after we left the next day to read off the brochure the story of the castle ghost; a former prince that haunts the night with a dagger in hand after having been murdered by his personal guard for stabbing a guest and raping his wife. While Kasey says that she is glad she stayed in a real haunted castle once and doesn't need to do it again, I loved spending the night in a real castle (haunted or not) and would do it again any time!

On Tuesday morning, after the sun was up and Kasey felt more comfortable exploring the castle, it was time for breakfast in the old soldiers' quarters and then our private tour. Since the castle was not stroller friendly, Kasey carried Clara in the chest carrier while we were escorted by a friendly hotel concierge who was wearing a tuxedo (at 9:00 a.m.). I wanted some candid shots of us on tour in the castle so, without anyone even noticing, when we entered a new room I would quickly set up the camera on a tripod in the corner and press the timer button.

When we were reviewing the photos from the trip, Kasey looked confused and asked who had taken these pictures. Since we were all in them, attentively listening to the concierge, she said it looked like we had been followed by a ghostly paparazzi the entire time!

We left relatively early after the tour to resume our route to Genoa, Italy, Monaco and then to Cannes in France. We would have needed to drive through Italy for another two hours before reaching Genoa. I felt much more comfortable with the idea of finding my way around Italy since I could speak some Italian and understood even more. Pretty soon after leaving the castle, we were driving through a valley with many fortresses that we could see from the highway. Being on a tight schedule, and having just spent the night in a castle, we did not feel compelled to stop. However, we found it unsettling to think how unsafe it must have been to live in a time when all these fortresses were necessary.

Upon entering the city of Torino, we got lost right away. I had not anticipated that the roads in Italy would be quite so different from anything else we had experienced so far. I had planned to take a different route to Genoa and the maps I had drawn were now useless. Although I was able to ask and get directions in Italian, the street signs (when there at all) were so confusing that it took us over an hour to leave the city. Other roads were just as challenging. I really missed having a GPS then. When we finally made it to the intersection where we would have turned to go to Genoa, we had already been driving for about three hours. Even though Clara was quite content with the driving around, Kasey and I were beginning to tire, and since I had been to Genoa once before, Kasey and I decided to skip it altogether, eat lunch and go directly to Monaco.

We did not linger in Monaco. With it being so small, we just drove around and felt satisfied. We continued toward Cannes where we were looking forward to resting in the hotel. We found it quickly and liked its location very much. The night was serene and cool so we went for a stroll, had dinner nearby out in the open, and went to bed earlier than usual. The next day, we needed to be in Barcelona by 2:00 p.m. for me to check in to work. We left early, but not before enjoying the treat of having breakfast on the rooftop of the hotel while viewing the sunrise over the city skyline and the Mediterranean. We arrived at our apartment just in time for me to start my work day with a conference call where I would get to "complain" with two other people in the office that I was a little tired because I had just arrived from having had breakfast in Cannes. Needless to say, I received no sympathy.

Outside the Lines

"Not all those who wander are lost." — *J.R.R. Tolkien*

There was a time when it was completely reasonable for people to expect their children to grow up, study, live and die in the same town as their parents. Parents thought that they would work in the same profession until retirement and so on. For a while now, it has been common in the U.S. for children to go to college in another state and most likely get a job and settle in a completely different place from where they grew up. More and more, people are having two or more careers in their lifetimes and moving several times across state lines seeking better opportunities. In pursuit of the American Dream, people now often work in several companies, get second careers, move to different states and adapt to different cultural and corporate environments. In Europe, the same forces are at play, except that people can now move across national borders and into cities with truly different cultures and languages.

During our travels in Europe, we carried our passports whenever we intended to cross into another country, although we never used them. All of the countries we visited were part of the Schengen Area—named after a village in Luxembourg where a deal to eliminate border checks was signed in 1985. This area is a group of 26 European countries (and growing) that have abolished passport and immigration controls at their common borders. When renting a car, they sometimes asked us if we were taking it out of the country, but they had no restrictions other than offering an additional insurance that would cover towing service outside of Spain. Since most countries are also using the euro, driving across countries is very much like driving across state lines in the U.S. One may see the old border crossings, but they are generally unmanned. If police are there at all, they just wave you in. We were absolutely fascinated by the ease with which one could drive (or move) into another country. Languages and customs would change immediately after crossing the imaginary lines we call national borders, but the general systems that make up the European Union remained the same. In each major city we visited, we saw people speaking many different languages. Some were visiting for sure, but many were living and working, and making these cities their new homes. These foreigners did not consider themselves immigrants, nor would the locals refer to them as such. They were just fellow Europeans born somewhere else. It was the same way a New Yorker is not considered an immigrant in Florida, but just a fellow American from a different state. No matter how many times we crossed national boundaries, we continued to be amazed at the truly international nature of today's Europe.

After moving to the U.S., while still trying to learn English and adapt to my new life in Colorado, I started remembering the many classmates and friends that I had growing up whose parents were Italian, Portuguese, Spaniard, German, Greek, Palestinian, French or Chinese. I never thought of my friends as foreign; they were just kids, like me. Their parents, though, did look very foreign to me. I remember the times when I would visit their homes and find myself surprised to share strange foods that I did not eat with my family. I would notice my friends' parents speaking to them in languages I did not understand, or treating them in ways that seemed a little odd. Sometimes, after Christmas or summer breaks, my friends would tell stories of vacations in faraway places where people ate, acted or dressed differently. These people were their friends and family, and my friends understood and enjoyed it all just as much as being home. As a child—more interested in games and school—I didn't think much of it at the time. But once I was in a foreign country, learning a new language, and adapting to a different culture, I was the one having the immigrant experience and I was the foreigner. I started thinking more and more about those early memories and found it curious how instead of relating to my contemporary classmates and friends, in many ways my current life and experiences had more in common with that of their foreign parents.

In 1908, oil was discovered in Venezuela. In just 20 years, the small South American country became the world's largest oil producer and exporter, second only to the United States. The bonanza created by the oil boom was accompanied by very open immigration policies. Living standards and opportunities were rising rapidly and pretty soon were much better than in many countries in Europe and Latin America. Immigrants started arriving in large numbers. In the late 1940s, Venezuela also aided displaced European refugees that could not, or would not, return to their homes after the devastation of World War II.

Immigration continued unabated for decades and Venezuelans were certain that their country was the richest and most desirable place to live in the world. But then, the unthinkable happened. Oil prices plummeted and foreign reserves started to dwindle. The country was forced to devalue its currency on February 18, 1983. This infamous day lives in the country's collective memory as Black Friday. The following Monday, the market crashed. The country fell into an abrupt and intense economic depression that brought about massive inflation, unemployment, and finally, political instability. Immigration came to a complete halt.

For the following 20 years after Black Friday, Europe and the rest of Latin America steadily improved while Venezuela continued to decline. In the 90s, rumors started circulating that the immigrants were starting to go back to their countries of origin. I remember a friend in middle school who always got perfect grades in English class because, somehow, she already spoke English. After finishing the school year, she did not return and I was told that she had moved "back" to the U.S. The following year, another close friend of mine was also gone; he had moved to Portugal. Another had moved to Italy, and others had gone to Spain, Germany, and so on. These stories of missing friends and neighbors became more and more common.

Venezuelan pride was deeply wounded by the realities of the crisis. The idea of immigrants leaving the country was perceived as rejection and even ingratitude, which was just another offence the still shocked society could hardly bear. Most people refused to believe the rumors and outright rejected the idea that anybody could have a better life anywhere else. They would say that the crisis was temporary and that all they needed was a new government with an honest and strong leader who could put the country back on track. They would insist that anyone who left would surely regret it and be back soon enough with their tail between their legs.

TV news reports started talking about the best college graduates leaving the country with job offers in Europe, Canada, Australia and the U.S. In the midst of the crisis, a newly elected government launched a massive nationalistic media campaign to fight what the news outlets were now calling a "brain drain." I could hear the resentment when people talked about it. Somehow these countries were stealing the most promising youth and with them the country's future. A government sponsored marketing campaign was launched aimed at convincing the youth that the country needed their talents to solve the temporary crisis. People desperately wanted to believe that with its internationally acclaimed beauty queens, great baseball players and wonderful weather, Venezuela remained the best place to live on earth. With its vast oil and mineral reserves, their country would always be the richest in the world. The country just needed a new generation of smart and honest people to be elected who would fix the economy.

This media campaign was only successful in making typical food and folkloric music popular again. But it also had the unintended (or not) effect of spreading the notion that those leaving were some kind of traitors that did not love the country. They would naturally take their life savings with them and this "fleeing capital" was equated to stealing the nation's wealth. The government eventually passed laws to stop people from being able to buy foreign currency. The economic crisis getting worse year after year eventually led to the beginning of a social breakdown with sporadic street riots, rising crime rates and even two consecutive failed military *coup d'états*. Although in retrospect, it is clear that I had plenty of reasons to leave, the national mood was still one of hope.

At that time, though, I already had dreams of traveling abroad and found it exciting to be on my own in new places and around people that I knew little or nothing about. While I was also a descendant of immigrants to Venezuela, my most recent foreign roots went back three generations to Italy, and the culture, the language and the family connections had been completely lost to me. After having traveled to Miami on several occasions, I had my sights set on South Florida;

however, my best friend had gone to Colorado to study English for a year before entering college. After visiting him in Colorado, he convinced me (rightly or wrongly) that Denver, being in the heartland, was the best place to learn English and assimilate the American culture. Eager to explore new frontiers, I decided to move there. My decision to leave the country was met with strong criticism from friends and acquaintances. My family's opposition was unrelenting. I was 19 years old when I decided to sell all of my possessions and leave the country before the end of the year.

A full decade after I left, foreign embassies in Venezuela started having long lines of young people applying for naturalization documents based on their parents' or grandparents' nationality. All of a sudden, people I had always known as proud Venezuelans, and who had criticized my decision to leave, were turning into Italians, Portuguese, Spaniards and Greeks. The grown Venezuelan children of immigrants were leaving for their parents' homelands in search of better opportunities. The last thing these parents wanted for their kids was for them to be immigrants as well. Never did these parents think that the rich, welcoming, tropical paradise, with the largest oil reserves in the world, would be in a state so dire that their own children would want to go back to the very countries they came from.

Many who did not have recent European ancestry started looking into getting student and immigration visas to Canada, Australia and the U.S. Immigrants from other Latin American countries started leaving as well. It looked like anyone that could get out, would; it looked like an exodus.

While I witnessed these events from afar, I still felt sad for so many people that were about to take part in the immigrant experience. Being exposed to different customs and ideas, looking at the country where I grew up from the outside and seeing the rest of the world through different lenses completely changed my life for the better and I would not trade it for anything. Nevertheless, the immigrant experience is far from a cakewalk. The misadventures of moving to a new country, losing everything and everyone one knows, having the need to learn a new language and adapt to different laws and customs, all while making a living, is not something I would recommend to anyone. With everything I gained from these very challenging experiences, I still wish I had acquired these multicultural skills at a slower pace, with the competent guidance and support of loved ones and at a younger age when learning would have been far easier.

I realize now how fortunate all those children of immigrants that I had known in my childhood were. They had grown up bilingual and bicultural from an early age without any effort or sacrifices on their part. They are perfectly comfortable in either their birth country or their parents'. They don't have an accent in either language and are never foreigners in either place. Their experience moving to a country different from that of their birth, although challenging as well, would be quite different from that of their parents' (and mine). They already spoke the language of their parents' country, had family roots, shared the culture and had dual citizenship.

While I was still studying English in Denver, I started to meet many exchange students attending college and even high school. Their parents had the vision (and the means) to enable them to live abroad and learn another language. From an early age, they had been exposed to different environments through extended vacations in different countries. They were not struggling with the *immigrant experience*. On the contrary, they enjoyed and embraced with excitement the newness of their surroundings and quickly adapted and excelled in their new environment. I decided then that this was what I truly wanted for my children.

Some countries that 30 years ago were great economic powers, are today in decline, while others that were relatively undeveloped, are today's fastest growing economies. The most successful and resilient corporations of today are multinational. Doing business all over the world, they need an executive work force able to handle different world markets. There is no way of knowing what the world will look like 30 years from now. But, if the past is any guidance, the sure thing to expect is even more change and more globalization. Being flexible, speaking another language and being comfortable in different cultures is only becoming more and more valuable over time. In some professional areas, these multicultural skills are no longer just a plus, but as much of a requirement as having a higher education.

I would like our children to be ready for the new flat world where our life's destiny is not only determined by the boom and bust cycles of one's place of birth, but also by events that happen on the other side of the planet. Speaking other languages, having a global view and a multicultural perspective will go a long way in preparing them for whatever the future holds. I would like their opportunities not to be limited by the ever changing economic, social or political realities of any particular country at any particular time. Just as today many people within the U.S. or within Europe need to move to different cities to attend the best schools or secure the best jobs, I want our children to be well prepared to move to different countries or even another continent if they ever have the need or just the desire.

I don't know if our children will decide to go into business, politics, medicine, the arts, science, ministry or sports, or if they will join the Peace Corps. But, no matter what they decide to do with their lives, I hope that having personal international experiences will open doors for them, or at the very least, give them a better understanding of the global events that affect us all, regardless of where we happen to live.

At Home in Barcelona

Family Values

"Price is what you pay. Value is what you get."
— Warren Buffett

Kasey's and my parents were not happy about having to wait so long to meet their new granddaughter. We would not get back to Florida until the very end of September and although we had plans to go visit Kasey's parents in S.C. during the first week of October, Clara would already be two months old. With me already going back to the office every day, Kasey would only have a couple of weeks to be with Clara by herself before returning to work in November. My parents were also dying to meet the baby, but it did not seem like we would be able to host them until December.

I should mention here that in my parents' world, it is not worth traveling overseas unless they stay at least an entire month. Staying in a hotel is completely out of the question since "we are family." And, as they would have been coming to meet their grandchild, they would have wanted to stay in our place all day. With me going to the office for work, it would have been left up to Kasey to entertain my non-English speaking parents while also taking care of our newborn in our small two-bedroom condo. They would have taken the suggestion that they stay less time, or in a hotel, as the final nail in the coffin of me kicking them out of my life. I know this because I have tried it before.

My parents already feared that with their grandchildren being born overseas and growing up in the U.S., they would rarely get to see them; my children would only speak English and would never get to know their *abuelos*. For us to rush to see Clara's American grandparents, while my parents had to wait until she was four months old, would make them feel left out of our lives. With Clara being their first grandchild, it seemed like all their fears were coming true.

Therefore, I devised a plan for them to meet their granddaughter right before we went back to the U.S. This visit would only be for a few days instead of a full month, they could stay in a hotel because our one-room rental was too small and they could claim to be the first grandparents to see the baby. Since both of Kasey's parents had declined our invitation to visit Spain, they could not even be jealous. While my parents had been to the U.S. many times to visit us, since we were in Europe, I thought that they could also get a different and interesting trip out of it. It was the perfect plan.

I told them over the phone that we would pay for the trip for them to come meet Clara and they were elated. I made arrangements for them to come to Barcelona for five days. I was hoping to find a hotel close to our place, but my parents are obsessed with what they call "value." That is, they should never, nor should anyone else, pay more for something than what *they* think it is worth. They were planning to stay with us to not have to pay for the hotel. Much to their displeasure, I explained to them that our place was too small to host anyone and that I would find and pay for a hotel room near us. Since we were staying by the beach in the middle of the summer, all the hotels nearby were booked and condos nearby were expensive and quite small in typical European fashion. I knew that they would ask me how much I paid for the hotel and I started stressing about finding something they would consider a "good value." The best I could do was a hotel 15 minutes away by subway. In Caracas where they live, they take the subway all the time and I thought that this would be familiar to them. My parents had made an international trip at least once a year for the past ten years (to visit us in the U.S.). They had also taken a European tour 20 years ago and a cruise through the Caribbean. Last, but not least, they spoke Spanish, so I thought they would be quite comfortable visiting us in Spain.

I was completely wrong. I told them about my plans and they were quite excited until the day I bought the tickets and booked the hotel. Immediately thereafter, they panicked. They started having all kinds of worries that I could never have imagined; things that they were hearing in the news about the debt crisis in Europe and how the continent was falling apart. As they started telling people they knew about their upcoming trip, all kinds of incredible warnings about Spain started pouring in about street protests, xenophobia and economic upheaval. According to one "authority," they would also need a "letter of invitation" from us to be allowed into the country. Without it, they were sure that they would be turned back upon arrival at the airport. They insisted that I go to the police station in Spain and request this letter (never mind that even if such a document existed, I was a tourist myself and would have had no right to "invite" anyone to Spain). No amount of explaining on my part would satisfy their concerns and after several arguments over the phone, I finally had to just tell them that the airfare and hotel were paid for and that I was too busy working full-time and taking care of my wife and newborn to sort out every urban myth they had ever heard.

Two weeks before we were due to fly back to Florida, my parents finally arrived in Barcelona without any problems. I went to pick them up at the airport and after they checked in to their very nice hotel (which they considered too expensive) we headed to our apartment for them to finally meet Clara. I was eager to show them the beautiful city of Barcelona including its subway, and yet, somehow on the subway ride to our place, only the large distance between their hotel and our apartment was worth discussing.

When we finally arrived at our apartment, my Dad was so anxious to meet Clara that as Kasey opened the door, he just exclaimed, *"al fin"* (finally), and took Clara from Kasey's arms before she could even say *"hola."* After a few minutes of gushing over Clara, they finally remembered to properly greet their granddaughter's mother as well. After commenting on how expensive and small our place was, they finally concluded that we could not have hosted anybody else there and that it was better for them to stay in a hotel.

I had hoped to show my parents around town and suggested that they come to our place every morning to go from there. Even though they are used to taking the subway in their home city, the idea of taking the subway in Barcelona and walking the three blocks to our place was too daunting for my Mother. She was terrified that she or my Dad would get lost in the city, despite the fact that the directions were extremely easy and they could ask anyone for help since they spoke Spanish. My Dad said that he could do it and they started arguing with each other. Soon, I realized that I would have to go pick them up and drop them off at their hotel every day. Other plans I had to rent a car for a weekend trip to Navarra quickly got canceled as well when I realized how uncomfortable they seemed to be in a foreign country.

We did manage to go to several places and festivities around town and my Dad finally got comfortable enough to ride the subway back to the hotel by himself the very last day (after drinking a few glasses of wine at our neighborhood festival). My Mom did also mention after going back to Venezuela that her misconceptions about Spain had completely changed and that the news reports and the things that people say have to be taken with a grain of salt. While I remember that week as being full of stress, they now speak about it as an interesting, fun trip where they got to explore Spain practically on their own.

Although I should have, of course, booked a better, closer hotel for them and paid much less for it.

Keys for Successful Travel

"Before anything else, preparation is the key to success."
— *Alexander Graham Bell*

We (or I should say Erick) only got locked out twice during our trip. As previously noted, the first time was in Mornas, France. We arrived in Mornas late in the evening, well after dark. Our hotel was in a striking location. It was just at the foot of a cliff that had an illuminated medieval fortress on top. Otherwise, though, we appeared to be in the middle of nowhere. Erick really likes fortresses. I find them a little creepy. I am also not a fan of suits of armor or any other symbols of medieval warfare. As Erick has already explained how well our hotel check-in went, I will not elaborate on that, except to reiterate that although I am normally a reasonable person, he is correct that I was not crazy about the large suit of armor that was stationed on the landing just outside our room. Once we got into our room, Erick left to go and find some food. As it was late, I fed Clara and laid her down. As I drifted off to sleep myself, I could still hear cheerful voices coming from the lounge downstairs.

The next thing I knew, I was awake and it was totally silent. The lights were dim, Erick was missing and I had no idea what time it was. Then I heard a faint thump. In my half-asleep state, it sounded like something hitting the window. I thought it must have been my imagination playing tricks. Then I heard it again. Now I was a little concerned because Clara and I were alone in this seemingly out of the way place. Thump. I finally walked over to the second story window and then I heard Erick. "Kasey!" He was yelling and whispering at the same time. "I'm locked out." Of the hotel? How do you get locked out of an entire hotel? "Come down and let me in," he said.

So with Clara snoozing in my arms, I crept out of the room. The hallway was now barely lit and with the suit of armor waiting for me on the stairs, it could have been the opening scene of any horror movie. I was concerned that I may not even be able to get out. I didn't have a key to the front door of the hotel. I made my way downstairs and over to the door. Thankfully, I could unlock it. As I opened the door to look for Erick, two dogs came running at me. In addition to suits of armor, I have an irrational fear of all dogs: large, small, yappy, it doesn't matter. I am the woman that all dogs chase because they instinctively know they can make me quake in fear. I slammed the door afraid these may be guard dogs or that they may charge inside. Finally, I saw Erick walking towards me and still talking, sort of, in really broken French to a man at the outer gate who seemed really annoyed. It was understandable as it was well after midnight now. Erick and I returned to our room where we laughed at his misadventures and enjoyed our sandwiches which were (appropriately?) stuffed with French fries. I also took the opportunity to read the bedside guide for additional hotel rules, just in case.

The second incident occurred one evening while Erick's parents were visiting when we were all distracted as we were leaving our Barcelona apartment. I was carrying Clara and I assumed that Erick had the keys, but he was busy talking to his parents about whether or not our dinner had been a good value and walked right out without them. Until then, I don't think either of us even realized that we could get locked out of our place. I thought we had to lock the door from the outside. I guess I was wrong. As soon as we got downstairs and discovered that no one had any keys, Erick set out for the management office that was a few streets away leaving Clara and me alone on the side street with his parents. After what seemed like way too long, and me having exhausted my capacity for small talk in Spanish (when we got married, Erick's Mother liked to joke, to the initial shock of her friends, that she and I were "not on speaking terms"), I told them that I was going to the office to see what was going on. I found Erick and he informed me that he was waiting on a locksmith.

When I returned to the apartment door, I did not see either of Erick's parents. Concerned about how we would find them if they had gone missing, I walked around the block to see if they were nearby. I found them both standing on the other side of the building staring up at the balconies. In the 15 or so minutes since I left, they had apparently devised a plan. Erick's Father began explaining. From what I thought I heard, he seemed to think we should "just" have someone (for example, Erick) go to a higher floor balcony and then climb down the outside of the building (five stories up) to our balcony and let themselves in through the sliding glass door. Had I understood that right? He seemed very serious. Erick's Mother was nodding her head in agreement. Although I was pretty sure there was no misunderstanding, I decided to act a little confused as I was not sure where to begin about why I thought this was a bad idea. There was certainly no urgency though since it was clear they had no volunteers. Thankfully, Erick returned just a few minutes later. His Father, still intent that we should not bother to pay a locksmith (I guess he didn't see much value in that), again explained his plan to Erick. From the look on Erick's face, I had understood just fine. Erick made it clear that no one would be climbing the outside of the building. About an hour (and 50 euros) later, we were back in the apartment for take two. We left again—both sets of keys in hand.

Let the Festivities Begin

"One does not leave a convivial party before closing time."
— Winston Churchill

The night before we were scheduled to return to the U.S. was extremely emotional for me. This was no doubt compounded by the fact that we had only recently returned from our longest and most ambitious international road trip, and had been hosting Erick's parents for several days amidst the largest and most energized festival Barcelona has to offer called *Les Festes de la Mercè* (in Catalan) or *Fiestas de la Mercè* (in Spanish). And believe me, to say it is Barcelona's best is saying a lot. I don't know if it is a fact, but much like I've read that the Inuit have dozens of words for snow, and have heard it joked that Brazilians know the difference between a beach and a *beach*, I wouldn't be surprised if there were dozens of words for "celebration" in Catalan.

The city itself has year-round festivals and events, but we really got lucky with our timing. In fact, in hindsight, we felt a little like Forrest Gump stumbling upon incredible historic sites and events in the most unexpected ways. From the wine festival in Olite, to UNESCO World Heritage sites, which were previously unknown to us, we kept finding extraordinary places in the most accidental manner. Even the clinic where Clara was born, which we initially chose simply because it was listed on our insurer's website, turned out to be the birthplace of several members of the Spanish royal family!

We arrived in Barcelona just weeks before Spain won the World Cup and ended up our time just after the *Mercè* Festival. Neither of us is a major sports fan, but since I knew we'd be there during the World Cup finals I started reading up on the games and teams before we left Florida. It was exciting to watch as Spain kept winning in each round and when we arrived in Spain, it was clear that soccer (or *fútbol*) was in the air. The Spanish team was only a few victories away from winning the whole thing and the entire country was watching. We watched the games on TV and I noted how much more exciting the Spanish speaking announcers were than their English counterparts. "*GOOOOOOOL!*" they would scream when anyone scored. It really transformed soccer watching into a completely different experience! We also tried to imagine how loud the vuvuzelas (the long plastic horns that had become a trademark of the South Africa World Cup) must have been in person. Even on TV, the stadium sounded like an enormous swarming bee hive. One evening, when Erick was on his 6:00 p.m. "lunch" break, we could see a game being played on a big screen in the upper room of the upscale pizza joint across the street from our balcony. So we headed over to have a drink and get in the spirit. The game was being showcased on a screen enclosed by an ornate gold frame as though it was an enormous piece of fine Italian art. I thought it added a nice sense of occasion and it certainly captured the mood.

We experienced the final game between Spain and the Netherlands with locals at another neighborhood restaurant while enjoying a giant seafood paella (more about those later) and Erick, at least, a pitcher of sangria. In hindsight, we should have made reservations, since virtually any restaurant with a TV filled up way before game time. We got one of the last tables just under the screen. The game went into overtime without a single point being scored and the anxiety in the room was palpable. Then in the final minutes, Andrés Iniesta scored for Spain and in an instant became a national hero. With that winning goal, the city exploded with street parties and chants of "*somos campeones*" (we are champions). What an introduction for us! We too went out into the streets and followed the crowds to the Christopher Columbus monument near the water. Fans were climbing the statute and cars were parading around the streets horns honking and flags waiving. I don't think anyone missed out on this celebration. (Well, except for that lonely group of fans down the street at the Dutch bar).

Speaking of sports, just down the beach from our apartment was an area of town that had been rejuvenated by the 1992 Barcelona Olympics. All along the *Port Olímpic* area of the beach there is a two tier row of restaurants and night clubs that would give Miami's famed South Beach a run for its money. A visitor walking along the upper boardwalk might be enticed to enter one of these venues via the rather non-descript "cubes" that dot the area. From the topside, these look almost like large one-room block construction houses. But inside, each cube has a distinct decor and a staircase leading down to the water level interior of a chic hotspot. You can find all kinds of music, cuisine, and if you're interested, even an ice bar, where you can don a rented polar jacket and go inside for a really cool drink. This area also, of course, has lots of delicious choices for traditional Spanish and Catalan dining. Erick and I, not really into clubbing on this trip, took advantage of the opportunity to eat!

One evening not long before Clara was born, we went in search of an authentic Spanish paella. Paella is served in a large round pan and usually consists of rice, vegetables, and either some type of meat or seafood. That night we found exactly what we were looking for. We chose one of the many open air restaurants on the beach that was advertising a special. After the first course of appetizers (bread topped with a delicious tomato paste), we were certain that the main dish must be on its way. We were shocked then when three more dishes were brought out before the enormous seafood paella. We thought we must have misunderstood the deal, but we were not complaining! Although stuffed, I could not resist when the server also brought out *crema catalana*, a dessert very similar to (if not identical to) *crème brûlée*. And all this (including a bottle of wine for Erick) for only 15 euros each! That night I really tested the limits of pregnant eating (so much for watching my weight), but I enjoyed every bite.

Another favorite weekend morning activity for us also involved the local cuisine. We loved to stroll over to the historic Gothic part of town and find a small plaza where we could people watch and feast on *tapas*. *Tapas*, which can be hot or cold, and can be simple or sophisticated, encompass a wide variety of appetizers that can be found in *tapas* bars throughout Spain. The ingredients vary and in most places you can survey all the choices before selecting those that suit your palate. The buffet style service encouraged newcomers, like us, to sample all kinds of new flavors. Erick, who while traveling in other countries, has been known to slam on the brakes whenever he sees a roadside stand with an unidentified fruit, particularly enjoyed these treats. I have also read that the serving of *tapas*, rather than an entire meal, was designed to facilitate conversation, which in our experience certainly seems to fit the culture. Some bars have restaurant style seating while others have only cocktail party style tables so that guests can circulate while they enjoy a light meal. As for us, we always enjoyed the food and the ambiance, so much so that Clara's first restaurant experience was at a favorite *tapas* bar situated in a small plaza near our home.

In addition to all of our eating, to be sure we didn't miss anything (which I finally admitted was impossible in Barcelona) I tried to keep up with the schedule of local events. Two weekends after Clara was born, she and I were both feeling well and I saw on my unofficial calendar of things-to-do that there was a festival going on in the *Gràcia* neighborhood. Each neighborhood (or *barrio*) has its own festival at a different time during the year, but from what I had gathered, this one was supposed to be one of the most elaborate. Not sure exactly what to expect, we packed up the stroller and headed over to the subway to find out. We went midday and soon discovered that this was an around-the-clock event. Each street in the *barrio* chooses a theme and then competes to have the best decorations. Block after block we were amazed at the detail and creativity of each competing street. Much of the décor was made from recycled materials that it seemed the residents had saved for this very purpose. The locals were hanging out in chairs and tables set out in the street sharing meals and no doubt preparing for the evening festivities of live music and dancing. Children, some of whom were in different team costumes, were running around the streets participating in a scavenger hunt which required them to perform all kinds of silly tasks. Everyone, whether young or old, seemed to be enjoying themselves. I was impressed at the level of coordination this all must have required. It was a real inspiration. What a way to get to know your neighbors!

That day, Erick and I also showed our inexperience as new parents. While we were out strolling around, Clara had a seriously stinky diaper. There was no obvious bathroom in sight and certainly not one where there was going to be a place to change her. Uncertain about our choices, we entered a small bar/café. The bathroom was tiny and there was no surface where I could imagine putting her down. Seeing our concern, the ladies working there graciously offered to let us use the top of a large cooler in the back of the bar. They assured me that it wouldn't be the first time! I took Clara back, spread out her changing pad and then one after another, each of the women in the restaurant came back to coo at little *Clarita*. Shortly thereafter, it finally occurred to Erick and me that we could just change Clara in the stroller which would lie completely flat. This turned out to be a very useful revelation. From that day forward, Clara was able to be a bit more discreet and we were freed from the constraints of a changing table!

Barcelona is also the capital of Catalonia, an autonomous region in the northeast of Spain. Although September 11th is a date that is now seared in the minds of many for tragic reasons, that date also marks the National Day of Catalonia. Catalan people can be found in Spain, France and parts of Italy and some eight million people speak the Catalan language (although many are multilingual, speaking other local languages, such as Spanish, French or Italian). Since the history of the region is long and complicated, I won't get into the specifics here, but suffice it to say that Catalans are a distinct group and there is increasing support in the region for independence from Spain. Catalonia is governed in part by its own *Generalitat*, which includes a parliament and local president, and which has made many decisions that show that Catalonia is distinct from Spain. For example, while we were there the region voted to ban bull fighting, a sport that it quintessentially Spanish. In fact, the enormous bull fighting ring in the center of Barcelona has since been converted into a really cool commercial center with shops and restaurants. There remains controversy, however, over whether the region should actually be permitted to split from the country. On the National Day, Catalan flags are waived, some of which have a star which indicates that the bearer supports independence. Others, without the star, simply seem to be showing a sense of local pride.

On Catalonia's National Day, we were out exploring the city with Clara when it became obvious that there was an event going on nearby. I knew about the holiday, but I had no idea what it might entail. We went in the direction of the music and came upon a large parade being held in support of Catalan independence just as it was reaching its final destination. This was not a riot scene or anything remotely like it. It was a festive party with little kids in strollers carrying toy drums. There was a platform at the end of the street where speakers were getting geared up for a rally and we watched as people placed wreaths at the foot of a monument that commemorates a centuries old battle. We saw both types of Catalan flags on display at the event. Of course, the speeches were being given in Catalan so we could not completely appreciate the message, but the scene appeared to be calm, well-organized and joyful.

One thing that everyone seemed to agree on, though, and that became almost comical to us, was the city's obsession with the cleanliness of its public spaces. Near our apartment, we were fascinated each night as a veritable army of workers and trucks emerged around midnight to comb the beaches and clean them for the next day. Erick also tells me that one evening when he was out late on an errand near Barcelona's famous *Las Ramblas* pedestrian thoroughfare, he witnessed some late-night partygoers duck behind a kiosk to avoid getting drenched by the street sprayer that was cleaning up after the busy day. We could not help but laugh then, when literally just feet behind the National Day paraders, followed a large team of neon green outfitted municipal workers sweeping up the street! They had wasted no time. Apparently, in Barcelona, demonstrations are permissible, celebrations welcomed—but cleanliness is indeed next to Godliness!

As I mentioned, at the end of September, the city kicks off the *Mercè* Festival, which is held in honor of the *Mare de Deu de la Mercè*, the patron saint of Barcelona. This festival goes on for an entire week and involves basically non-stop activities for any taste. To prepare for what I understood would be an overwhelming list of choices of things to do, I attended the free weekly culture class at my language school during the week preceding the festival. There I learned about several of the must-see events and activities. One event that I found most curious was where a group of people known as *castellers* would gather to build human castles. One afternoon while Erick's parents were visiting, I insisted we go and check this out. As we approached a large central plaza we encountered throngs of people who also had the same idea. We could not quite reach the plaza itself for the crowds and had to stand on a side street and look in. This turned out to be just fine however, as the castellers can rise up to eight human "stories" above the crowd! Neighborhoods apparently create teams that prepare for this event in which each team wears a different matching color. The heaviest castellers stand in a large circle with their arms linked to create the "ground floor." Then, increasingly smaller and younger castellers climb up the outside of the growing tower until the final team member, usually a five year old child (now required to wear a helmet), climbs all the way to the top and throws up one hand to signify that the tower is complete! When the little hand goes up the crowd cheers and goes wild with applause in appreciation. The youngest castellers then seem to almost slide down the outside of the tower safely back to the ground. The whole thing is quite a spectacle and is not to be missed if you visit during the festival. Other teams don't form circles at all, but simply stack themselves four individual people high on each other's shoulders and then actually parade through the crowd!

In addition to the castellers, throughout the week, there are other parades featuring *gigantes* which are oversized effigies of kings, queens and nobles, and fireworks each night on the beach. These are not novice fireworks displays, and rival anything I have ever seen at a large U.S. city's Fourth of July celebration, except that these went on for several nights in a row! As an aside, just after we arrived in Barcelona, on the Fourth of July, we spotted a man with a lone sparkler in the distance. I can only imagine that he was a U.S. expat determined to celebrate Independence Day despite being abroad. While we enjoyed walking out to the beach to see the fireworks, when we were in the apartment, the noise echoed off the surrounding buildings creating thunderous booms. At first, I was concerned about Clara, but we would cover her ears and she never seemed to mind. Like us, she seemed to be soaking up the energy of the city.

One evening after Clara and I had been walking around a carnival style fair that was also going on in our neighborhood, Erick returned from sightseeing with his parents. He explained that the *gigantes* roaming all over town had kept him from being able to get back home to start work on time. I couldn't wait to hear him explain that to his employer. I thought "the giants kept getting in my way" sounded about as good as "the dog ate my homework!" Erick encouraged me to go and see if I could catch the tail end of the parade. I transferred Clara to Erick and his parents, grabbed my subway ticket and a few euros, and headed out solo eager to see what was happening just a few blocks away.

By the time I reemerged from the metro, the *gigantes* were long gone, but there was a mass of people in the plaza where a large stage had been set up, which looked big enough to host a rock band. Assuming that there would be a concert, I decided to hang around and see. I went into a large sandwich shop on the side of the plaza where crowd control procedures had been put in place so that festival goers could efficiently secure a take-away dinner. I purchased my sandwich and headed up to the third level of the shop where I got a seat right beside a window. I now had a bird's eye view of the thousands of people and stage below. I tried to ask a lady nearby what everyone was waiting on, but all I could understand was that the "show" was about to begin. Great! I was excited to hear some live music. By then though it was dark out and there was no sign of any band. Then the show finally started. It was not on the stage as I had expected, but was instead taking place on the facade of the large government building that dominated the plaza. I guess you could call it a light show, but that really does not do it justice. It was one of the most unique displays I had ever seen. The projectors made the building appear to melt and shake and would then shift gears to show silhouetted men and women jumping from window to window in a mischievous dance. The building was transformed into an old school boombox that pulsated with rhythm and then into bubbles that appeared to fly away. The show went on for almost an hour and was by far the coolest part of the festival for me. I just wish I had better words to describe it and that Erick had been there to enjoy it with me. Even baby Clara might have enjoyed the lights and the music. Although I am sure we only scratched the surface of what the *Mercè* Festival had to offer, we certainly had a blast just trying to keep up.

And just when I thought the city couldn't party any more, our local neighborhood, Barceloneta, was getting geared up for its own drum choir festival. This is exactly what it sounds like. In a seemingly spontaneous (but certainly coordinated) fashion, drum corps of a dozen or so people would assemble in the streets of Barceloneta and parade around throughout the day and night performing rhythmic shows for all to enjoy. One day when Erick was trying to participate in a conference call for work, one such drum band emerged just below our balcony and started their set. While the band was drawing a crowd and Clara and I were enjoying the free in-house entertainment, Erick was huddling in the hallway trying to get some quiet. Again, I am sure some things are just inexplicable to a conference room full of executives half a world away. As part of the festivities, the residents just one block over strung lights and decorations from one building to another to make it appear as though the street below had a ceiling of plastic wrapped candies. The neighborhood set up tables and a stage for live music and late-night dancing. It was in this environment that we began packing our bags and preparing to leave.

Farewell

"Isn't it funny how day by day nothing changes, but when you look back everything is different?" — C.S. Lewis

Our last night in Barcelona had arrived. After packing and cleaning, we were everything but ready to leave. While Clara was sleeping in the bedroom, Kasey and I were talking on the balcony looking down the street. We were appreciating the meaning of the last three months and the effect that it had had on us, all that we had learned and how we had gotten so much closer. We were so happy with our lives, and so excited to have a healthy beautiful baby. We were filled with a sense of accomplishment and gratitude for having Clara and having fulfilled our dream. Yet, we were also sad; sad to see the end of a chapter in our lives that had been so rich, intense and exciting. We had felt so alive and made so many memories in the last three months that it felt like it had been years. The little apartment felt like home now. We had our first child in that place. We had seen Clara smile for the first time there. We had cried, worried and laughed together there. We would miss this time in our lives very much. We would miss the beach, the subway, the streets, the local market, the girl that sold us our bread each day and the ladies that sold us ham and cheese. We would miss the guy that Kasey terrorized in the pharmacy, the nice old ladies in the neighborhood (even the one that smacked me) and our church friends. I would miss our weekends driving to strange lands in little rented cars. As we were pondering these thoughts on our little balcony while looking at the moon, Kasey started crying. Then she started laughing, surprised to be crying. I completely understood. I felt the same way. This chapter in our lives was ending and we realized that it would not return. It would now be a memory. We would never be new parents again. Clara would never be our newborn baby again.

We were not sad to just leave a place behind. One can always return to a place. We were sad to leave a time behind.

Coming to America

Seven Wonders

"Oh, the Places You'll Go!" — *Dr. Seuss*

The next morning we awoke before the sun came up to catch a cab to the airport. Driving down the dark streets through our neighborhood, I remained nostalgic from the night before. Once we got to the airport, we were offered the opportunity by the airline to be bumped to a flight the next day. At first, we thought they were offering cash to any passengers who would accept as well as food and lodging accommodations for the night. We seriously considered it, but later realized they were offering airline "dollars" instead of hard currency. In hindsight, maybe we still should have taken it. After all, it could have funded future adventures. But, at least for me, having already said my goodbyes and having packed our bags, I was prepared to go. I was also a little anxious about flying with Clara. She had done great on our road trips, but we were not sure how she would react to eight hours in the air. It turned out to be a breeze.

The plane was large enough to have three seats in a middle section as well as additional seats on either side of each aisle. Since we knew we would have Clara on the flight, we had booked seats in the middle of the cabin—the ones with the wall in front of them instead of another seat. The airline offered an in-flight bassinet that could be attached to the wall for Clara to sleep in. Once we took off, the stewardess attached a small metal frame to the hooks on the wall and we placed a blanket over its mesh bottom. It also had a breathable mesh cover that could be secured over the top of the bassinet to keep Clara safely inside in case of sudden turbulence. I thought this was a great idea and Clara did agree to sleep in it for at least half of the flight. The rest of the time, she hung out with mommy and daddy or on the bathroom changing table that was also conveniently located near our seats. She did not have any problems with the flight and many passengers commented that they did not even realize a baby was onboard. Our arrival in the U.S. marked Clara's seventh country in just two short months. She was already a world traveler in the making.

Apparently, when we landed, I did not call Mom quickly enough to let her know we were safely back. We had been picked up at the airport by some good friends in Florida and we were busy introducing them to Clara. As she sometimes does when worried about my brother or me, Mom called Dad to see if he had heard from us. She said that she would have thought we would have called by then. Dad responded, true to form, "I would have thought she would have had her baby in the *United States*, but that didn't happen either." So much for total acceptance of the Big Idea, I guess.

Nothing Could be Finer

"In my mind I'm going to Carolina.
Can't you see the sunshine; can't you just feel the moonshine?"
— James Taylor, "Carolina In My Mind"

Just over a week after our return to Florida, we traveled to South Carolina to visit my family. I went up first with Clara since Erick had gone back to work and he joined us on the weekend. Clara, already a champ at flying, slept peacefully the entire two hour flight in the baby carrier I was wearing on my chest. When I arrived at the small Greenville/Spartanburg airport, I could see Mom, Dad and my stepmother (Grandma Lynn-Lynn, Papa John and Mama Dee, respectively) waiting by the glass divider for their first real life glimpse of Clara. As soon as we got into touching range, Mom burst into tears—again—but this time out of joy. She kept saying how she didn't think she would do that. We all shared a hug and Clara woke up just in time to get caught up on lots of kisses. We spent the next week visiting and getting to know my brother and sister-in-law's second daughter, who had been born just weeks after Clara. The grandparents reveled in having all of their girls in one place.

Reflections

If You Want to Make God Laugh

"A man's heart plans his way, but the Lord directs his steps."
— Proverbs 16:9

They say that there are three things everyone should do to achieve a full life: (1) plant a tree; (2) write a book; and (3) raise a child. A few years before Clara was born, a small brown box arrived at our doorstep. I took it to the kitchen and opened it on the counter. Inside there was a tiny, frail, weed-like plant and a small typed note that said, "Help me! I've been in this box for three days with no water!" Erick explained that this was the "tree" he had ordered online. In addition to having always wanted to give every opportunity to his children, as I learned back then, Erick also loves trees and dreamed of planting some himself. This tree was supposed to grow at an extraordinary rate of over 12 feet per year so it was an excellent choice. According to its promo, you could measure the progress daily. Erick lovingly planted it in our yard and we waited to witness the miracle. Unfortunately, the very next day I looked out the window and saw it all slumped over on the ground. Perhaps we should not have planted it in the direct July sunlight? Neither of us claims a green thumb. We brought the tree inside and Erick, already showing his nurturing side, began trying to nurse it back to health in an orange juice carton. He would move it from the kitchen to the window to try to give it just the right conditions, and then tried to plant it in the yard at least two more times, but it was just too late. The damage had been done and we had to sadly say our goodbyes to the tree. As we finalize this book, although we still have hopes for another tree in the future, we are pleased that we are at least making progress toward the other two goals.

In addition to working our way through these three things, though, Erick and I are also in search of a more *deliberate* life.

We are in many ways conditioned to go through the motions of life without really appreciating the choices we make for ourselves and for our families. A culture of busyness gets in the way of mindfulness regarding our own values and goals. It is too easy to just go with the flow. Of course, we cannot control our every eventuality, and as the saying goes: "If you want to make God laugh, just tell Him your plans." But we must have a say, and we must at least be *aware* of our decisions. After all, if we do not make plans for our lives someone else, be it an employer, a marketer, a family member, or some other interested party, certainly will. I, for one, do not want to leave it up to chance.

During our time in Europe, I felt that we were practicing the skill of deliberate living. It was easier while we were away, because when you know that you only have a limited time in a place or with certain people you are inclined to make the most out of it. That was certainly true of our time in Barcelona. Since we knew we only had three months abroad everyday became an adventure. We were so *conscious* of our time that it seemed to slow down for us during our stay. I have often heard people talk about how quickly time flies by as a person gets older and I wonder if this is not in large part the result of our lives simply becoming too routine. In contrast, in our experience while we were away, even little things became more interesting (and challenging) because our environment was new and different. As a consequence, even with moments of exhaustion and anxiety, our first months with Clara were even more intensely joyful. The reality for all of us of course, is that our time is *always* limited. We do not know how much we have. I fear that I, like so many others, have been taught to survive life, to wait until "someday" and hopefully wind up with "enough." While it is certainly prudent to consider one's future, I do not want to put off dreams just to realize one day that it is too late. The risk is simply too great.

Finally, although the word "crisis" may have a negative connotation, it is actually defined as a crucial stage or turning point. In this sense, my time with Clara in Spain was certainly a crisis in my life. Fortunately, during such a time we can more easily make changes. For me, understanding that I wanted to live deliberately was the most important change I could have made, and it is one lesson I look forward to sharing with my children.

After all the worries and warnings expressed by all kinds of people when they heard of our plans to have our first baby born overseas, I reached the conclusion that I would be more private in any future plans we may have. I still expected a lot of questions after we returned and we were eager to share the wonderful stories and experiences we had during those three months. It was amazing to notice, though, that the same people that were the most worried about every possible bad thing that could happen seemed barely interested in knowing about the great things that did happen.

Fear and anxiety are very powerful emotions when embraced, and allowed to grow they can become permanent advisors inside our heads. The more we listen to these advisors, the stronger their voices become, until eventually they get all of our attention. If there is nothing to fear or worry about there is simply nothing to say, nothing to ask. Very little room, if any, is left for curiosity, learning or even joy to celebrate everything that is great.

The optimistic people that were excited for us from the beginning were eager to know how everything went and wanted to hear all the details. Some of these people suggested that we write this book and their excitement encouraged me to start this work. I hope that writing the memories of this adventure will help us cast aside the voices of fear and anxiety that so often hinder us from living life to the fullest and that ultimately, we are encouraged to continue turning our dreams into achievable goals by asking: *What would it take?* My goal is that this exercise will be only the beginning for us to continue living what we have come to call *a deliberate life*.

Marriage Counseling

"Never fear quarrels, but seek hazardous adventures."
— Alexandre Dumas, The Three Musketeers

It is also important to note here that after the fact, and upon reflection, Erick and I did question whether we were crazy to put our marriage to the test in all the ways we did on this trip. Having a baby can be stressful enough all by itself and I'm sure it has led many otherwise happy couples to counseling. The fact is people can no longer ignore their differing views on all kinds of things once they have a child together and many don't realize it until that day comes. And there we were, me pregnant (and later with a newborn), in a foreign country where I didn't speak the language, in a tiny apartment, with Erick working full-time late into the evening and making regular weekend road trips into neighboring countries where neither of us spoke the language. Given the potential for marital strife, I cannot in good conscience recommend this to everyone. That is not to say that Erick and I did not have our disagreements, both before and after Clara's arrival, but we are both big on communication and we talk *a lot*. If this idea intrigues you, I suggest you do your research, really consider whether this works for both you and for your partner and remember that communication and flexibility are key!

I once heard from motivational speaker Tony Robbins, that a life worth living is a life worth recording. Neither Kasey nor I had written a book before we set out to write this one. With that in mind, I will say that writing this book was an adventure of its own. It was a new and very different experience for each of us. It required many hours working together and separately. If our experiences on our trip had not been enough to bring us closer, writing this book forced us to bring to light many of our most private reflections. This helped us get to know ourselves and each other even more deeply.

Story Telling

"If history were taught in the form of stories, it would never be forgotten." — Rudyard Kipling, The Collected Works

When we learned that I was pregnant, Erick immediately wanted to share the news with friends and family, but I was hesitant. I thought I wanted to wait a while to be sure everything would be okay. But then again, as my husband pointed out, weren't these the people who would be there for us should there be a problem? And of course, we can never know the future, so what was I waiting for. This was not something to hide, but I have always been a very private person, tending to reserve for myself my thoughts and dreams. In college, I dropped a public speaking course because the first assignment was to bring in an item that explains who you are. Mind you, I withdrew not because I had a fear of public speaking (I later became a lawyer), but because I simply did not want to share that much about myself. Likewise, it was very difficult for me to share our plans for a maternity leave abroad and I found myself waiting until the very last minute to tell people. By the time we returned, however, I could not wait to share our experience.

Of the struggles I faced on this unique journey into motherhood, some of the hardest were not caused by real challenges at all, but were instead the result of my harboring the concerns of others. With everything from breastfeeding to travel, I discovered that my stress was often simply a manifestation of someone else's worry. The gradual understanding that these worries, which were not even my own, could have held me inert was at once disconcerting and liberating. As a result, so much of my journey to Spain had nothing to do with geography, but instead with freeing myself from fear and convention in order to live a more deliberate life. That is the story I most wanted to tell here. Openly conveying the emotions surrounding this time in the history of our family—the apprehensions and the excitement—makes the process of writing this book a personal success. I am realizing more and more that a satisfied life is one which is shared with those around you. It is for this reason that I wanted to once again step out of my comfort zone, overcome the fear that kept me from finishing my public speaking course and share this story for my children and for myself. The writing of this book has not been a final chapter for us, but has instead punctuated the end of one journey and made way for the beginning of another.

www.ingramcontent.com/pod-product-compliance
Lightning Source LLC
Chambersburg PA
CBHW030439290526
45786CB00001B/366